# Tobacco Cessation
## A Practice Manual for
## Primary Care Physicians

# Tobacco Cessation
## A Practice Manual for Primary Care Physicians

Edited by
## Rajmohan Panda
## Manu Raj Mathur

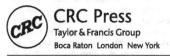

**CRC Press**
Taylor & Francis Group
Boca Raton London New York

CRC Press is an imprint of the
Taylor & Francis Group, an **informa** business

CRC Press
Taylor & Francis Group
6000 Broken Sound Parkway NW, Suite 300
Boca Raton, FL 33487-2742

First issued in paperback 2021

ISBN-13: 978-0-367-13324-5 (hbk)
ISBN-13: 978-1-03-208427-5 (pbk)

This book contains information obtained from authentic and highly regarded sources. While all reasonable efforts have been made to publish reliable data and information, neither the author[s] nor the publisher can accept any legal responsibility or liability for any errors or omissions that may be made. The publishers wish to make clear that any views or opinions expressed in this book by individual editors, authors or contributors are personal to them and do not necessarily reflect the views/opinions of the publishers. The information or guidance contained in this book is intended for use by medical, scientific or health-care professionals and is provided strictly as a supplement to the medical or other professional's own judgement, their knowledge of the patient's medical history, relevant manufacturer's instructions and the appropriate best practice guidelines. Because of the rapid advances in medical science, any information or advice on dosages, procedures or diagnoses should be independently verified. The reader is strongly urged to consult the relevant national drug formulary and the drug companies' and device or material manufacturers' printed instructions, and their websites, before administering or utilizing any of the drugs, devices, or materials mentioned in this book. This book does not indicate whether a particular treatment is appropriate or suitable for a particular individual. Ultimately it is the sole responsibility of the medical professional to make his or her own professional judgements, so as to advise and treat patients appropriately. The authors and publishers have also attempted to trace the copyright holders of all material reproduced in this publication and apologize to copyright holders if permission to publish in this form has not been obtained. If any copyright material has not been acknowledged please write and let us know so we may rectify in any future reprint.

---

### Library of Congress Cataloging-in-Publication Data

---

Names: Panda, Rajmohan, editor. | Mathur, Manu Raj, editor.
Title: Tobacco cessation : a practice manual for primary care physicians /
[edited] by Dr. Rajmohan Panda, Dr. Manu Raj Mathur.
Other titles: Tobacco cessation (Panda)
Description: Boca Raton : CRC Press, [2020] | Includes bibliographical
references and index. | Summary: "Cessation of tobacco use is the need
of the hour given that it is the single largest cause of disease and
premature death in the world. This book covers epidemiology and risks,
user classification, nicotine replacement therapy, pharmacological aids,
behavioral modification, and patient counseling techniques, and
personalized action plan development"-- Provided by publisher.
Identifiers: LCCN 2019035075 | ISBN 9780367133245 (hardback ; alk. paper) |
ISBN 9780429025884 (ebook)
Subjects: MESH: Tobacco Use Cessation | Primary Health Care
Classification: LCC RA1242.T6 | NLM WM 290 | DDC 613.85--dc23
LC record available at https://lccn.loc.gov/2019035075

---

Visit the Taylor & Francis Web site at
http://www.taylorandfrancis.com

and the CRC Press Web site at
http://www.crcpress.com

# Contents

Foreword, vii

Preface, ix

Acknowledgments, xi

Editors, xiii

Contributors, xv

Abbreviations, xvii

CHAPTER 1 ▪ Introduction                                                    1

MANU RAJ MATHUR

CHAPTER 2 ▪ Tobacco and Health                                              9

SANDEEP MAHAPATRA AND KUMAR GAURAV

CHAPTER 3 ▪ Theories of Tobacco Addiction                                  23

SONU GOEL AND SUSANTA KUMAR PADHY

CHAPTER 4 ▪ Behavioral and Psychological
Approaches for Tobacco Cessation                                           39

SONALI JHANJEE

CHAPTER 5 ■ Pharmacological Approaches for
Tobacco Cessation 57

BINOD KUMAR PATRO AND SURAVI PATRA

CHAPTER 6 ■ How to Develop a Tobacco Cessation
Center 71

RANA J. SINGH

CHAPTER 7 ■ Patient Follow-Up 85

VIKRANT MOHANTY

CHAPTER 8 ■ Evaluation of Cessation Practices 95

RAKESH GUPTA

CHAPTER 9 ■ Frequently Asked Questions 101

INDEX, 107

# Foreword

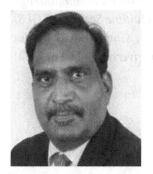

EVERY YEAR, LAKHS OF NEW TOBACCO USERS TASTE TOBACCO for many reasons, whether to appear mature, to influence someone, for fun, or to just try it and soon become addicted. Expenditure incurred on the treatment of tobacco-related diseases and the serious health consequences have always drawn the attention of the Government of India to curb it. Even people who know and have suffered from the deadliest outcomes of tobacco still use it. A majority of users want to quit but do not know how to. The withdrawal symptoms always create trouble in leaving the vicious circle of nicotine addiction. Physicians and other health care professionals need to be aware and well-trained in tobacco quitting processes.

This book *Tobacco Cessation: A Practice Manual for Primary Care Physicians* is written with precise scientific procedures for tobacco cessation treatment protocols. The book further deals with the necessary aspects of tobacco cessation, namely, theories of tobacco addiction, behavioral and psychological approaches for tobacco cessation, pharmacological approaches for tobacco cessation, patient follow-up, evaluation of cessation practices, and so forth. There is no doubt that this book will definitely increase the knowledge of physicians in tobacco cessation programs and provide a better understanding. I appreciate the sincere attempt of the editors in presenting this very valuable book, which is a welcome addition for physicians and private practitioners as well as for readers and medical students.

**Raj Kumar, MD**
*Professor, Department of Pulmonary Medicine*
*Head, National Centre of Respiratory Allergy,*
*Asthma & Immunology*
*In-Charge, National Tobacco Quitline Services (TQLS)*
*Government of India*
*Vallabhbhai Patel Chest Institute, University of Delhi, Delhi*

# Preface

TOBACCO USE IS THE SINGLE LARGEST CAUSE OF DISEASE AND PREMATURE DEATH IN THE WORLD. It is the only consumer product that kills half of its regular users—tobacco is directly responsible for 5.4 million deaths, annually. In India, tobacco is responsible for over eight lakh deaths each year. Studies worldwide indicate that people who quit using tobacco live longer than those who continue with its use. Cessation of tobacco use is therefore the need of the hour apart from various community awareness and socio-legal initiatives primarily aimed at prevention.

Health care professionals play a pivotal role in providing cessation services. This manual has been developed to increase the knowledge of clinicians in tobacco cessation and treatment services and can easily be integrated in their day-to-day practice. The manual has been developed with input from national and international experts who work in tobacco cessation and consists of evidence-based cessation methods for health care professionals. The manual, through various chapters covers all the necessary elements of tobacco cessation, namely, tobacco epidemiology and risks, benefits of quitting, models for behavior change as applied to tobacco cessation, the necessary elements for documentation in the patient tobacco cessation profile, behavioral modification techniques, classification of tobacco users according to their stage of change (5 stages: pre-contemplation, contemplation, preparation, action, and maintenance), nicotine replacement therapy, pharmacological aids for cessation, patient counseling techniques, and the development of a personalized action plan.

The module is self-explanatory and will help professionals working in primary care facilities and other health care settings to deliver evidence-based tobacco cessation services in their routine clinical practice. We hope that the doctors will find this manual a useful resource to strengthen their day-to-day practice, provide effective cessation services, and help reduce the catastrophic health and economic loss caused as a result of tobacco use.

**Rajmohan Panda**
**Manu Raj Mathur**
*New Delhi, India*

# Acknowledgments

THIS MANUAL WAS PREPARED BY THE PUBLIC HEALTH FOUNDATION OF INDIA (PHFI) by a team of cessation experts and researchers.

We express our sincere gratitude to the Government of India and the state governments of Odisha and Rajasthan for their partnership in implementing the SCCoPE (Strengthening Cessation Capacity of Primary Care Professionals) project.

Special thanks to Dr. Hayden McRobbie, Professor of Public Health Interventions, Health and Lifestyle Research Unit, Queen Mary University of London. We would also like thank Dr. Sonu Goel for his thorough review of the manual, and for his comments, corrections, and suggestions.

We would like to express our appreciation to Dr. Divya Persai for proofreading the manual and Dr. Deepti Nagrath for her technical input. We express our gratitude to Mr. Awadhesh Kumar and Mr. Amit Singh Rajawat for their support in publishing this book.

We would like to also express our indebtedness and gratitude to all the authors without whose dedication and support, the production of this manual would not have been possible.

We are also very grateful to Professor K. Srinath Reddy, President, PHFI for his support and guidance.

# Editors

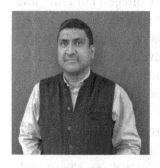

**Rajmohan Panda, MD, MPH,** is a senior public health specialist and additional professor at the Public Health Foundation of India (PHFI). He has a Global Health Leadership master's degree from Emory University (Atlanta, Georgia), a certificate from the Global Tobacco Control Leadership Program from Johns Hopkins, and a Public Health Leader Implementation research certification in Noncommunicable Diseases (NCDs) from Emory University. He has worked on diverse public health issues, such as nutrition, maternal child health, tobacco control, and in the design of health sector reforms for universal health coverage. He has worked widely across India with various stakeholders including state health departments, the Ministry of Health and Family Welfare—Government of India, the Gates Foundation, USAID, UNICEF, DFID, and Wellcome Trust and Medical Research Council UK. His interests include translational research, and he has been involved in leading studies for evidence generation for more meaningful health outcomes. Dr. Panda's work focuses on academic case studies on pertinent public health issues ranging from maternal child health to examining systems capacity in chronic and noncommunicable diseases. His interests include building capacity in tobacco cessation in primary care in the country and he has worked in several states to design and evaluate tobacco cessation training programs in primary care and corporate settings.

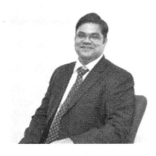

**Manu Raj Mathur, PhD**, is a dental surgeon with a PhD in epidemiology and population health from the University College London and a master's in public health with a specialization in dental public health from the University of Glasgow (UK). He is currently head of the Health Policy and is additional professor at the Public Health Foundation of India (PHFI), New Delhi. He was a recipient of the prestigious Fogarty International Clinical Research Scholarship in 2010–2011, a Wellcome Trust scholarship for his doctoral studies in 2009, and another Wellcome Trust Mid-Career Fellowship to undertake work on psychosocial determinant inequalities in oral health in India. His areas of expertise include operations and health systems research and health promotion. Dr. Mathur has worked on many projects funded by the Government of India, WHO, BMGF, USAID, and NIH in the past and is currently leading large-scale projects from MRC UK, Global Bridges Consortium, the Government of India, and the Rockefeller Foundation. He has authored many high-impact peer-reviewed journal articles and is the author of many chapters in multiple global health books. He holds an honorary clinical lecturer position at the University College London. In addition, he teaches various courses offered at different institutes of PHFI on health promotion, principles of public health, epidemiology, health systems, and tobacco control modules.

# Contributors

**Kumar Gaurav**
MLE Specialist
Concurrent Monitor and
    Learning Unit
Bihar Technical Support
    Programme
CARE India
Bihar, India

**Sonu Goel**
Additional Professor of Health
    Management
School of Public Health
Post Graduate Institute of
    Medical Education and
    Research
Chandigarh, India

**Rakesh Gupta**
Senior Advisor and President
Rajasthan Cancer
    Foundation
Jaipur, India

**Sonali Jhanjee**
Professor
All India Institute of Medical
    Science (AIIMS)
New Delhi, India

**Sandeep Mahapatra**
Associate Epidemiologist
Decision Resource Group
Bengaluru, India

**Vikrant Mohanty**
Associate Professor
    and HOD
Maulana Azad Institute
    of Dental Sciences
New Delhi, India

**Susanta Kumar Padhy**
Additional Professor of
    Psychiatry
All India Institute of Medical
    Sciences (AIIMS)
Bhubaneshwar, India

**Suravi Patra**
Additional Professor
Department of Psychiatry
All India Institute of Medical
  Sciences (AIIMS)
Bhubaneswar, India

**Rana J. Singh**
International Union against
  Tuberculosis and Lung
  Disease (The Union)
New Delhi, India

**Binod Kumar Patro**
Additional Professor
Department of Community
  Medicine & Family
  Medicine
All India Institute of Medical
  Sciences (AIIMS)
Bhubaneswar, India

# Abbreviations

| | |
|---|---|
| ANM | auxiliary nurse midwife |
| ASHA | accredited social health activist |
| CO | carbon monoxide |
| COPD | chronic obstructive pulmonary disorder |
| CVD | cardiovascular disease |
| GATS | Global Adult Tobacco Survey |
| HCP | health care professional |
| ICD | International Classification of Diseases |
| MI | motivational interviewing |
| nAChRs | nicotinic acetylcholine receptors |
| NCDs | noncommunicable diseases |
| NGO | non-governmental organization |
| NRT | nicotine replacement therapy |
| NTCP | National Tobacco Control Program |
| PAH | polycyclic aromatic hydrocarbon |
| PHS | public health services |
| SD | substance dependence |
| SUDI | sudden unexpected death in infancy |
| TB | tuberculosis |
| TCC | tobacco cessation center |
| TD | tobacco dependence |
| TSNA | tobacco-specific nitrosamines |
| VTA | ventral tegmental area |
| WHO | World Health Organization |

# CHAPTER 1

# Introduction

Manu Raj Mathur

## Objectives

The major objectives are to

- Learn about the burden of different forms of tobacco use

- Understand the importance of tobacco cessation and role of physicians

## Skill Sets You Will Acquire

You will be able to conceptualize

- The burden of tobacco use in India

- The importance of tobacco cessation services in India

- The role of health care professionals in tobacco cessation

## BACKGROUND

In India, every third adult consumes tobacco* which is an established major risk factor for noncommunicable diseases

---

* Tobacco use is a risk factor for six of the eight leading causes of death in the world.

(NCDs), leading to one million smoking-related deaths per annum. The death burden is expected to rise in low- and middle-income countries, like India, due to the current pattern and alarming rise in tobacco use.[1,2] There are 275 million tobacco users (111 million smokers) in India that mostly affect the vulnerable lower socioeconomic and rural populations (Figure 1.1).[3]

Tobacco use is classified under mental and behavioral disorders in accordance with the International Classification of Diseases (ICD-10).[4] Around 53% current smokers in India have either no interest in quitting or are undecided about their intention to quit. A slightly higher proportion (55%) of current tobacco users report no intention to quit. This clearly signals the need to fully utilize a range of cost-effective tobacco control approaches such as legislation, education, and cessation. A comprehensive tobacco control approach (Figure 1.2) will help reduce smoking prevalence and the associated morbidity and mortality in the long term. But, among these, tobacco cessation interventions will reap health benefits in the short term, leading to a reduction in near-term tobacco-related mortality and morbidity,[5-7] whereas others would take two to three decades.

Health care professionals have a role to play in all aspects of tobacco control, but their position naturally lends itself to "W," to *w*arn about the dangers of tobacco, and, "O," to *o*ffer help to quit.[8]

Since 2001, only 19 public tobacco cessation centers have been established in India.[9,10] Their establishment within the tertiary care health facilities gave only a limited access to tobacco users, particularly to those living in rural areas. They were also poorly accessed by youth.[11] These centers, therefore, could serve only 34,741 tobacco users during the first 5 years; a small fraction of tobacco users who made an attempt to quit.[11] The available manpower in these centers was also inadequate to serve the population of 20–40 lakhs (2–4 million). It is critical, therefore, to address the need for socially vulnerable groups with limited access to cessation service utilization by establishing countrywide tobacco treatment

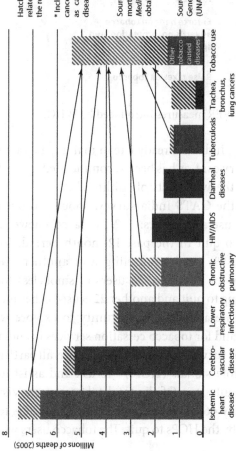

Hatched areas indicate proportions of deaths that are related to tobacco use and are colored to the column of the respective cause of death.

*Includes mouth and oropharyngeal cancers, esophageal cancer, stomach cancer, liver cancer, other cancers as well as cardiovascular diseases other than ischemic heart disease and cerebrovascular disease.

Source: Mathers CD, Loncar D. Projections of global mortality and burden of disease from 2002 to 2030. *PLoS Medicine*, 2006, 3(11): e442. Additional information obtained from personal communication with C.D. Mathers.

Source of revised HIV/AIDS figure: AIDS epidemic update. General, Joint United Nations Programme on HIV/ AIDS (UNAIDS) and World Health Organization (WHO), 2007.

FIGURE 1.1 Tobacco use is a risk factor for six of the eight leading causes of death in the world. (From *WHO Report on Global Tobacco Epidemic*, 2008.)

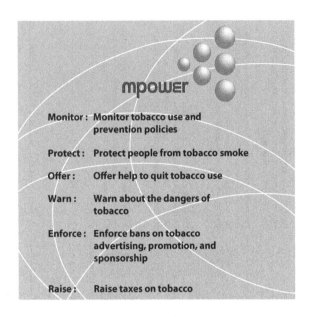

FIGURE 1.2    MPOWER measures introduced by WHO.

facilities. In a way, India is already late in making its provision at the level of primary care, as has been recommended by the WHO, with reference to the availability of quitlines.[12]

According to the GATS India survey, about two out of five current tobacco users (smokers: 38%, tobacco chewers: 35%) have attempted to quit in the past 12-month period. In 2010, among smokers, 9% used counseling and another 4% used pharmacotherapy for cessation. In users of smokeless tobacco, 8% used counseling to quit and another 22% used other methods. These facts indicate an ample opportunity to explore ways to improve the demand for tobacco cessation services in India.

The GATS India survey also reports that the overall participation of health care professionals (HCPs)—to ask and assist tobacco users to quit is quite low. Of the total tobacco users visiting a health facility, only 46% smokers and 27% of smokeless tobacco users were asked by the HCPs to quit. The tobacco users who were further assisted to quit was even lower. This raises concern about the capability of HCPs to intervene with tobacco users. A system-wide approach to tobacco treatment, at various levels of health care would greatly assist HCPs. This has yet to be addressed.

Empowering doctors to provide behavioral counseling details for the skills (counseling) needed for tobacco treatment is a challenge. The behavioral change theories (e.g., plans, responses, impulses, motives, evaluations [PRIME]) and techniques[12] are a cornerstone of tobacco cessation counseling and the application of these principles to tobacco cessation requires soft skills on motivating tobacco users to quit using tobacco. The traditional curriculum does not train HCPs in soft skills. Therefore, to deliver tobacco treatment optimally, the need to train all health professionals in acquiring the necessary soft skills for motivating people to quit using tobacco is critical and urgent.[13]

Counseling along with pharmacotherapy adds to the efficacy of the cessation of treatment. Their combined effectiveness is higher than their separate uses. In fact, together, they double the success rate for quitting smoking. However, this is not done routinely in India.

There is an urgent need to empower HCPs at all levels of health care on tobacco cessation approaches, including behavioral skills and pharmacotherapy through on the job training or a continuing education system in addition to its inclusion in the curriculum of doctors and nurses at the undergraduate level. Further, instead of being just theoretical, as is presently the case, through the training manuals available, it should be contextual, practical, and adaptable to the local needs. Unfortunately, there are only a few reports on tobacco treatment from India. Hence, an adaptation of the existing scientific knowledge to the vastly varied Indian context is another challenge. This manual, therefore, integrates the updated scientific knowledge about evidence-based psychological principles and the best practices in tobacco treatment, adapted to India with focus on their application in real-life situations.

**KEY MESSAGES**

- Tobacco use is an addiction, a mental and behavioral disorder that the country and the people of India cannot afford
- To quit, tobacco users will benefit from the assistance provided by health care professionals
- Although evidence of effective tobacco cessation interventions is mostly from a non-Indian setting, there is no reason to believe that these will not work in the Indian setting
- Health care professionals should
  - Warn the public of the dangers of tobacco use
  - Motivate and offer help to smokers to quit tobacco use

## REFERENCES

1. Jha P, Jacob B, Gajalakshmi V et al. A nationally representative case-control study of smoking and death in India. *N Engl J Med* 2008;358:1–11.
2. World Health Organization. *WHO Report on the Global Tobacco Epidemic—2011*. Geneva. WHO, 2011.
3. Ministry of Health and Family Welfare. *Global Adult Smoking Survey (GATS)-India, 2009–10*. New Delhi: Ministry of Health and Family Welfare, Govt. of India, 2010.
4. Hong Wang H, Sindelar JL, Busch SH. The impact of tobacco expenditure on household consumption patterns in rural China. *Soc Sci Med* 2006;62:1414–26.
5. U.S. Department of Health and Human Services. *The Health Benefits of Smoking Cessation: A Report of the Surgeon General*. Rockville, MD: U.S. Department of Health and Human Services, Centers for Disease Control and Prevention, Office on Smoking and Health, 1990.
6. Kulik MC, Nusselder WJ, Boshuizen HC et al. Comparison of tobacco control scenarios: Quantifying estimates of long-term health impacts using the DYNAMO-HIA modeling tool. *PLOS ONE* 2012;7(2):e32363.
7. Peto R, Lopez AD, Boreham J et al. *Mortality from Smoking in Developed Countries 1950–2000. Indirect Estimation from National Vital Statistics*. Oxford, UK: Oxford University Press, 1994.

8. WHO-MPOWER. http://www.who.int/tobacco/mpower/publications/en/.
9. Varghese C, Kaur J, Desai NG, Murthy P, Malhotra S. Initiating tobacco cessation services in India: Challenges and opportunities. *WHO South East Asia J Public Health* 2012;1(2):159–168.
10. Murthy P, Saddichha S. Tobacco cessation services in India: Recent developments and the need for expansion. *Indian J Cancer* 2010; 47:69–74.
11. Varghese C, Kaur J, Desai NG et al. Initiating tobacco cessation services in India: Challenges and opportunities. *WHO South East Asia J Public Health* 2012;1(2):159–168.
12. WHO. *Developing and Improving National Toll-Free Tobacco Quit Line Services*. Geneva: WHO, 2011.
13. Michie S, Churchill S, West R. Identifying evidence-based competences required to deliver behavioral support for smoking cessation. *Ann Behav Med* 2011 Feb;41(1):59–70. doi: 10.1007/s12160-010-9235-z.

# CHAPTER 2

# Tobacco and Health

Sandeep Mahapatra and Kumar Gaurav

**Objectives**

The major objectives are to

- Describe major health consequences of tobacco use
- Clarify common misconceptions held by tobacco users
- Explain the benefits of quitting tobacco use

**Skill Sets You Will Acquire**

You will be able to conceptualize

- A basic knowledge on tobacco use and its effects
- Myths and facts about tobacco use
- Benefits of quitting

## HEALTH IMPACT

Tobacco Kills up to Half of Its Users

As a leading cause of death and illness, tobacco kills around 6 million people who directly use tobacco (both smoking and

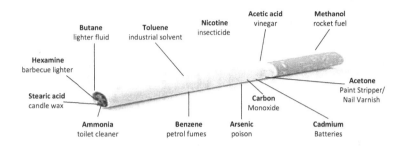

FIGURE 2.1    Major toxins in tobacco smoke.

smokeless) worldwide each year.[1] Secondhand smoke is also associated with health risks, resulting in more than six lakh premature deaths per year, worldwide. There is no safe limit for the use of any type of tobacco.[2,3] It is highly addictive and causes many serious illnesess.[4,5] In spite of its harmful effects, studies show that only a few tobacco users are aware of its risks to their health and the benefits of quitting. The majority know that tobacco use is harmful, but still they continue with its use. About 70% users desire to quit, but it requires assistance. Therefore, as health care professionals, we need to inform patients (and the communities at large) using tobacco about its harmful effects and benefits of quitting.

## Composition of Tobacco and Tobacco Smoke

Smoking is bad for health because tobacco smoke contains more than 7000 chemicals, of which at least 250 are known to be harmful, and approximately 70 are known to cause cancer (see Figure 2.1).[6,7] Although nicotine in very high doses can be lethal, the amount received by smokers does not cause significant harm to physical health—it does, however, keep them addicted to tobacco use.

## ADVERSE HEALTH CONSEQUENCES OF TOBACCO USE

There is ample evidence on the consequences of tobacco use on health. Figure 2.2 illustrates that tobacco use and secondhand smoke damage every part of the body.[2,3]

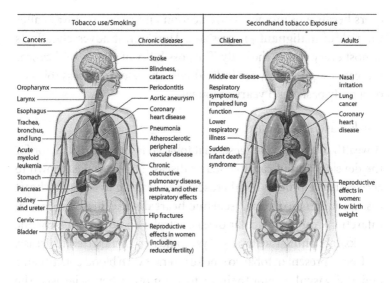

| Tobacco use/Smoking | | Secondhand tobacco Exposure | |
| --- | --- | --- | --- |
| Cancers | Chronic diseases | Children | Adults |

FIGURE 2.2 Diseases caused by tobacco use/smoking and secondhand smoke. (From the U.S. Department of Health and Human Services; *How Tobacco Smoke Causes Disease; The Biology and Behavioral Basis for Smoking Attribution Disease; A Report of the Surgeon General,* Atlanta, GA; U.S. Department of Health and Human Services, Centers for Disease Control and Prevention, National Center for Chronic Disease Prevention and Health Promotion, Office on Smoking and Health, 2010.)

The major health effects of tobacco use include: (A) cancer, (B) noncancerous lung diseases, (C) atherosclerotic diseases of the heart and blood vessels, and (D) toxicity to the human reproductive system.

## Tobacco and Cancer

Tobacco contains approximately 70 carcinogens that may induce or promote carcinogenesis.[2] Although nicotine itself is not carcinogenic, nicotine addiction is responsible for chronic tobacco use and exposure to carcinogenic substances. Many carcinogens, including polycyclic aromatic hydrocarbons (PAHs) and tobacco-specific nitrosamines (TSNAs), appear to cause cancer following metabolic activation. Cancer does not develop in all tobacco users because numerous detoxification and repair pathways alter the risk of malignant progression. However, it adversely affects almost every part of the body. The possibility of getting oral cancer increases significantly for individuals who use smokeless tobacco on a daily basis for 3 years or longer.

## Cardiovascular Disease

A wealth of evidence suggests that tobacco is a major risk factor for the development of cardiovascular disease.[8,9] Tobacco is known to accelerate the process of atherosclerosis, leading to coronary heart disease (angina pectoris, ischemic heart disease, and myocardial infarction), cerebrovascular disease (stroke and transient ischemic attacks), abdominal aortic aneurysm, and peripheral arterial disease.

Toxins present in tobacco smoke interact with blood constituents and the vascular endothelium to promote atherosclerosis, the primary pathophysiologic feature of cardiovascular disease. Atherosclerosis is characterized by the deposition of lipid in the arterial wall, fibrosis, and vascular thickening. Further exacerbating the atherogenic and thrombotic effects of tobacco on the vascular system are the physiologic demands on myocardial tissue resulting from an imbalance of oxygen supply and demand. Smoking may contribute to ischemia and precipitate acute events (myocardial infarction, unstable angina, and sudden death) in patients with atherosclerosis.

## Smoking and Respiratory Disease

Smoking has significant adverse health effects on the upper and lower respiratory tract system.[2,7] Smoking-induced respiratory disease is divided into two categories: acute (predominantly caused by infections) and chronic (disorders of the conducting airways and alveoli).

### Acute Respiratory Disease

Exposure to tobacco smoke incudes a variety of acute respiratory diseases affecting both the upper and lower respiratory tracts, which paralyzes cilia on columnar respiratory epithelium and compromises protective mucociliary transport host defenses and tars in smoke concentrate in pulmonary alveolar macrophages inhibiting the phagocytic activity of these cells. The net effect is reduced host defense against infections caused by respiratory pathogens.

*Chronic Respiratory Disease*
Infants exposed to maternal smoking in utero are more likely to have measurable evidence of impaired lung function, although the mechanism for this impairment is not known. Likewise, children, adolescents, and adults exposed to tobacco smoke are more likely to experience chronic respiratory symptoms (cough, increased phlegm production, wheezing, and dyspnea). Irritants and oxidant gases present in tobacco smoke are believed to worsen airway inflammation and exacerbate bronchial hyperresponsiveness. Due to the inflammation and damage to the pulmonary tissue, the airways narrow down, resulting in chronic obstructive pulmonary disease (COPD).

## Tobacco and Reproductive Health

Tobacco use is associated with numerous reproduction-related complications, including effects on fertility, pregnancy and pregnancy outcomes, and infant mortality.[2] Smoking leads to vasoconstriction and hypoperfusion at the site of placental implantation leading to necrosis, hemorrhage, and separation. Components in tobacco smoke might disrupt the cytokine system, impair reproductive tract immune function, or promote inflammatory processes leading to preterm birth. A dose-dependent increase is seen in the risk for preterm delivery in pregnant smokers. Nicotine-induced vasoconstriction in the placenta may induce preterm labor. Women who smoke during pregnancy are more likely to deliver infants with low birth weight (i.e., <2.5 kg). The risk of sudden unexplained death in infancy (SUDI) is higher among infants with mothers who smoke during pregnancy and among those who are exposed to environmental tobacco smoke after birth.

## SECOND AND THIRDHAND SMOKE

Smoking is a habit that causes mortality and morbidity in both its users and nonusers. It is simply because it can negatively affect each organ of the body. It is interesting to understand how tobacco smoke affects the nonusers of tobacco. There are 7000 chemicals in tobacco smoke (70 that we know cause cancer). When inhaled, the body quickly absorbs these 7000 chemicals, causing changes in body cells that can lead to cancer, heart disease, and other serious health issues. There is no safe level of exposure.

Tobacco smoke is placed into three categories:

- Firsthand smoke, which is inhaled by the smoker.

- Secondhand smoke, which is the smoke either exhaled by a smoker or released from the burning end of a cigarette.

- Thirdhand smoke, which is the tobacco smoke residue and gases that are left after a cigarette has been smoked.

### Secondhand Smoke

Secondhand smoke affects the respiratory system of nonsmokers through mechanisms similar to those by which tobacco smoke affects the airways and lungs of active smokers. However, since the levels of exposure are lower, the effects of secondhand smoke tend to be less severe.[1]

Secondhand smoke is further classified into sidestream smoke (the smoke that comes from the burning end of a cigarette) and mainstream smoke (the smoke exhaled by the smoker). Sidestream smoke makes up about 85% of secondhand smoke. It is made up of different chemicals than exhaled mainstream smoke because it burns at a lower temperature, and the burn is not as clean or complete. Secondhand smoke exposure affects an adult's heart and blood vessels instantly. Adult nonsmokers who live with smokers are at about 25% more risk of developing heart disease. Secondhand smoke causes lung cancer even in nonsmokers.

*Effects of Secondhand Smoke on Babies and Young Children*
Secondhand smoke is harmful especially for babies and young children as they are in their growing phase. Exposure to secondhand smoke may cause the following disorders:

- Low birth weight, which increases the chance of developing heart disease and type 2 diabetes when they grow up.

- A higher risk of sudden infant death syndrome (SIDS).

- Serious lower respiratory infections, such as bronchitis and pneumonia.

- Respiratory symptoms, including coughing, mucous, wheezing, and shortness of breath.

- More ear infections than in a child who is not exposed to secondhand smoke (they are also more likely to have tubes placed in their ears to drain the fluid caused by a high incidence of ear infections).

Moreover, children who suffer from asthma experience more attacks and these can often be more serious. Traces of cancer-causing toxins and other such toxins are found in the blood, urine, saliva, and the breast milk of nonsmokers, even after little exposure to secondhand smoke. Opening windows in buildings or traveling by vehicles does not protect one from the effects of secondhand smoke. This may get rid of the smell; however, it does not get rid of the cancer-causing toxins in the air. Only 100% smoke-free environments protect you from secondhand smoke.

*Effects of Secondhand Smoke on Adults*
Secondhand smoke also has detrimental and long-standing effects on adult nonsmokers as well. Some of them are

- Nonsmokers exposed to secondhand smoke commonly experience eye, nasal, and throat irritation.

- An elevated nasal ciliary beat frequency (a defense mechanism that transports secretions, particles, and other substances out of the nasal passages) comparable to smokers.

- A range of chronic and acute respiratory symptoms in nonsmokers are also associated with the exposure to secondhand smoke, such as cough, phlegm, and sputum production, wheezing, and shortness of breath, in people both with and without asthma.

- Secondhand smoke may also be responsible for causing the onset of asthma in adulthood, and for making the management of asthma more difficult. Evidence suggests that people with asthma have a small acute decline in lung function following exposure to secondhand smoke.

- Adults exposed to secondhand smoke have a higher likelihood of snoring, and are at a greater risk of experiencing respiratory complications during surgery involving anesthesia.

- Research suggests that exposure to secondhand smoke may cause an elevated risk of developing COPD, which is marked by permanent and progressive damage to the airways and airway sacs of the lung.[1] COPD results in reduced lung function that is largely irreversible.

Thirdhand Smoke
Thirdhand smoke is made up of the residue and gases of tobacco smoke, that

- Includes the gases that go back into the air
- Stays on surfaces and in dust after tobacco has been smoked

- Builds up on surfaces, furniture, clothing, drapes, and carpets
- Reacts with other elements in the environment to add to pollution

When tobacco is burning, it releases nicotine in the form of a vapor. This vapor attaches to surfaces such as walls, floors, carpeting, drapes, and furniture. Nicotine reacts with nitrous acid (one source of which is burning tobacco) and forms cancer-causing tobacco-specific nitrosamines (TSNAs). Nicotine can last for months on indoor surfaces. This means that these TSNAs are always being created. TSNAs are then inhaled, absorbed, or ingested. Anyone who smokes in any enclosed space (like a car or home) is exposing nonsmokers to TSNAs.

Children are more sensitive to being exposed to thirdhand smoke because they breathe near, crawl on, play on, touch, and even taste (because they often put their hands in their mouths) surfaces contaminated with tobacco residue. This adversely affects the pregnant woman and the fetus.

Experts on thirdhand smoke recommend 100% smoke-free homes and vehicles. They also suggest that replacing furniture, carpets, drapes, and so forth, can greatly reduce exposure to thirdhand smoke residue.

## MISCONCEPTIONS ABOUT THE HEALTH EFFECTS OF TOBACCO USE

There are a number of common misconceptions about tobacco use that may be used to justify ongoing tobacco use. These should be corrected with facts (see Table 2.1).

## BENEFITS OF QUITTING TOBACCO

Tobacco users should be informed that quitting tobacco saves lives and money. In fact, the benefits begin immediately and continue as long as tobacco users stay away from it (see Table 2.2).

Quitting tobacco can confer significant financial benefits also.[10,11] The money that a tobacco user spends can be saved

TABLE 2.1 Common Misconceptions about the Health Effects of Tobacco Held by Tobacco Users

| Myths | Facts |
| --- | --- |
| Low-tar cigarettes are safe to smoke. | There is no safe cigarette; a low-tar cigarette is just as harmful as other cigarettes. |
| Cutting down the number of cigarettes smoked will eliminate health risks. | There is no safe level of cigarette consumption. Smoking at even low levels is associated with adverse health effects such as acute cardiac events. |
| Only old people get ill from smoking. | Anyone who smokes tobacco increases their risk of ill-health. All age groups suffer short-term consequences of smoking. |
| Smoking relieves stress | Many smokers believe that smoking alleviates stress. However, this misattribution is due, at least in part, to the fact that smoking alleviates tobacco withdrawal symptoms that can feel like stress. The fact is that when smokers quit long term they actually become significantly less stressed than when they were smoking. |

if they quit. The financial benefits of quitting tobacco can be explained using a simple method as shown in Figure 2.3.

So, if you follow the aforementioned simple ways of briefing your patients and tobacco users, it could influence them to make an informed choice of quitting tobacco successfully. As a result, tobacco users will be spared of its risks and will add years to their life, regardless of the age at which they quit.

## CASE STUDY 1

When Ramesh was 16, his father—a cigarette smoker—died of lung cancer. Despite his loss, Ramesh started smoking 3 years later. Ramesh quit smoking at 34 years of age because he could not bear the thought of missing out on any part of his own daughter's life. Ramesh also had an emotional reason to quit smoking: as a teen, he lost his father to lung cancer. He knew that toilet breaks and car trips would tempt him, so he carefully planned quitting by using nicotine patches, walking, and friends' support. Ramesh hadn't thought

TABLE 2.2   Health Benefits of Quitting Tobacco

| Health Benefits |
| --- |

**1. There are immediate and long-term benefits of quitting for all smokers.**

| Timing since quitting | Beneficial health changes that take place |
| --- | --- |
| Within 20 minutes | Heart rate and blood pressure drop |
| 12 hours | The carbon monoxide level in blood drops to normal |
| 2–12 weeks | Circulation improves and lung function increases |
| 1–9 months | Coughing and shortness of breath decrease |
| 1 year | Risk of coronary heart diseases is about half that of a smoker |
| 5 year | Stroke risk is reduced to that of a nonsmoker 5–15 years after quitting |
| 10 years | Risk of lung cancer falls to about half of that of a smoker and risk of cancer of the mouth, throat, esophagus, bladder, cervix, and pancreas decreases |
| 15 years | Risk of coronary heart disease is that of a nonsmoker's |

**2. Benefits for all ages and people who have already developed smoking-related problems. They can still benefit from quitting.**

| Time of quitting smoking | Benefits in comparison with those who continued |
| --- | --- |
| At about 30 | Gain almost 10 years of life expectancy |
| At about 40 | Gain 9 years of life expectancy |
| At about 50 | Gain 6 years of life expectancy |
| At about 60 | Gain 3 years of life expectancy |
| After the onset of life-threatening disease | Rapid benefit, people who quit smoking alter having a heart attack reduce their chance of having another heart attack by 50% |

**3. Quitting tobacco decreases the excess risk of many diseases related to secondhand smoke in children such as respiratory diseases (e.g., asthma) and ear infections.**

**4. Quitting smoking reduces the chances of impotence, difficulty in getting pregnant, premature births, babies with low birth weight and miscarriage.**

*Source:*  Fact sheet about health benefits of smoking cessation—WHO.

about all the ways smoking hurt his daily life until he quit. After that, life started getting better quickly. Food tasted better. He had more energy and more confidence. And there was one big surprise. The money he saved from not smoking was absolutely great!

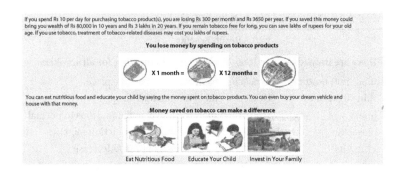

FIGURE 2.3   The financial benefits of quitting tobacco.

### KEY MESSAGES

- Tobacco is the single-most preventable cause of death globally
- Tobacco use and secondhand smoke damage every part of the body
- Tobacco imposes enormous economic costs on individuals, families, and the country
- Quitting tobacco saves lives and money
- Health care providers should assist tobacco users to quit the habit by explaining the risks of its use, and the benefits of quitting, supported by simple examples

## REFERENCES

1. Gajalakshmi V, Peto R, Kanaka T, Jha P. Smoking and mortality from tuberculosis and other diseases in India: Retrospective study of 43000 adult male deaths and 35000 controls. *Lancet* 2003;362:507–15.
2. Centers for Disease Control and Prevention. CDC TIPS Tobacco information and prevention source. Available from: http://www.cdc.gov/tobacco/, accessed on October 12, 2012.
3. U.S. Department of Health and Human Services. *How Tobacco Smoke Causes Disease: The Biology and Behavioral Basis for Smoking-Attributable Disease: A Report of the Surgeon General.* Atlanta, GA: U.S. Department of Health and Human Services,

Centers for Disease Control and Prevention, National Center for Chronic Disease Prevention and Health Promotion, Office on Smoking and Health, 2010.

4. *WHO Report on the Global Tobacco Epidemic*, 2008. The MPOWER package: www.who.int/tobacco/mpower/en/

5. Gender, Health and Tobacco, WHO 2003. www.who.int/gender/documents/Gender_Tobacco_2.pdf

6. European Union. Health effects of smokeless tobacco products. SCENIHR. Available from: http://ec.europa.eu/health/ph_risk/committees/04_scenihr/scenihr_cons_06_en.htm, accessed on October 15, 2012.

7. Ferlay J, Bray F, Pisani P, Parkin DM. *GLOBOCAN 2002: Cancer incidence, mortality and prevalence worldwide.* Lyon: International Agency for Research on Cancer (IARC) Press, 2004.

8. Benowitz NL. Cigarette smoking and cardiovascular disease: Pathophysiology and implications for treatment. *Prog Cardiovasc Dis* 2003;46:91–111.

9. Kamholz SL. Pulmonary and cardiovascular consequences of smoking. *Med Clin N Am* 2004;88:1415–1430.

10. Jena P, Das S, Khillar A. Expenditure in tobacco product: Using economy for advocacy. *Int J Tuberc Lung Dis* 2012;16(12):S256.

11. The health benefits of smoking cessation. DHHS Publication No. (CDC) 90-8416. Washington, DC, Department of Health and Human Services, 1990.

# CHAPTER 3

# Theories of Tobacco Addiction

## Sonu Goel and Susanta Kumar Padhy

### Objectives

The major objectives are to

- Explain the physiology of tobacco dependence

- Provide an overview of different theories of tobacco dependence

### Skill Sets You Will Acquire

You will be able to conceptualize

- Various theories of tobacco dependence

- Understand the basics of tobacco dependence

- Critically express the need for physicians to know about the theories of tobacco dependence

## INTRODUCTION

### What Is Tobacco Dependence?

Tobacco dependence (TD) is an addiction to tobacco products. The drug primarily responsible for tobacco dependence is nicotine; however, there are other substances in tobacco that contribute to tobacco dependence. The essence of drug dependence is loss of control over drug use. It is often mistakenly assumed that people with substance dependence (SD), including tobacco dependence, lack moral principles or willpower.[1,2]

### Is Tobacco Dependence Different from Other Substance Dependence?

The basic understanding of TD, according to the clinical diagnostic criteria in the ICD-10 International Classification of Mental and Behavioral Disorders, is similar to those of other substance dependence. However, there are some differences. For example, TD does not cause behavioral problems. Many individuals with TD who stop tobacco use do so without treatment. However, many who try will not be able to stop the long-term use of tobacco so stand to benefit from tobacco cessation treatment.[3,4]

### How Do We Understand the Process of Tobacco Dependence?

Figure 3.1 summarizes the process of TD, from the first time or the experimental use to regular use. Relapse is common, and so interventions to assist people to stop tobacco use often need to be repeated.

### Why Do Some People become Addicted While Others Do Not?

No single factor can predict whether a person will become addicted to tobacco. Risk for TD is influenced by a combination of factors that include individual biology, age, or stage of development and social environment. The more risk factors and less protective factors (see Figure 3.2) an individual has, the greater the chance that taking

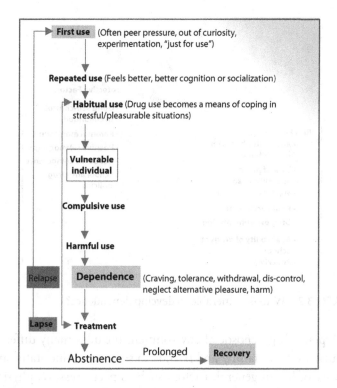

FIGURE 3.1   Process of tobacco dependence.

tobacco can lead to dependence.[5] For example, the genes people are born with, in combination with environmental influences—account for about half of their dependence vulnerability. Genetic and environmental factors interact with critical developmental stages to affect dependence vulnerability.[6] Although taking drugs at any age can lead to dependence, the earlier nicotine use begins, the more likely that it will progress to more serious abuse. Adolescents may especially be prone to such addictive behaviors because the brain areas that govern decision making, judgment, and self-control are still in the developmental phase. Additionally, gender, ethnicity, and the presence of other mental disorders (such as schizophrenia, bipolar disorder, depression, and anxiety disorder) may influence the risk of tobacco dependence.

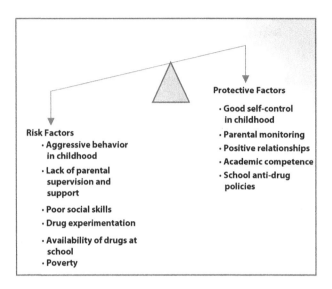

FIGURE 3.2    Who is vulnerable to develop dependence?

A person's psychosocial environment includes many different influences, from family and friends to socioeconomic status and quality of life in general. Factors such as peer pressure, physical and sexual abuse, stress, and quality of parenting can greatly influence the occurrence of tobacco abuse and the escalation to dependence in a person's life.[1,2,5–8]

## THEORIES OF TOBACCO DEPENDENCE

There are numerous theories propounded by various authors. However, for the sake of simplicity and better understanding, a few key theories are presented in this chapter.

### Psychodynamic Theories

According to the classic psychodynamic theories, substance use, including TD is a masturbatory equivalent (i.e., pleasure feeling). For some, TD is a defense against anxious impulses, or a manifestation of oral regression (i.e., dependency). Recent psychodynamic explanations theorize that an individual abuses a substance as a consequence of disturbed ego functions (i.e., the inability to deal with reality).[1,3,4]

## Theory of Learning and Conditioning

Occasional drug use or compulsive drug use is a behavior maintained by its consequences, mediated by a behavioral phenomenon called reinforcement. The stimulating effect of nicotine can produce improved attention, learning, reaction time, problem-solving ability, and better mood (i.e., positive reinforcement). Tobacco users also report that it reduces tension and low mood, and alleviates withdrawal symptoms (i.e., negative reinforcement). In some social situations, drug use can be reinforcing if it results in approval from friends or special status (positive reinforcement). Eventually, the paraphernalia (e.g., cigarette packs, lighters) and behaviors associated with tobacco use (e.g., drinking alcohol, socializing) can become secondary reinforcements, signaling the availability of the tobacco product.[1,3,4,9] In the presence of cues (internal/external), craving (a strong desire to consume tobacco products) increases. This phenomenon is called "cue conditioning." Tobacco users respond to the nicotine-related stimuli with increased activity in limbic regions of the brain, including the amygdala and the anterior cingulate.

Characters in the movies or television often show smoking as a part of daily life. These may attract vulnerable adolescents toward smoking as a desirable "grown-up" activity. Those children who are exposed to cigarette brand names through television are more likely to smoke by the phenomenon of "vicarious learning."[10] In vicarious learning, a "mental representation" for smoking, of the "television character"/"celebrity"/"brand ambassador," is formed, which gets activated when they are exposed to cues.

Other learning mechanisms play a role in dependence or relapse. For a long time after tobacco withdrawal, the individual exposed to environmental stimuli previously linked with tobacco use (e.g., watching a friend light a cigarette, a colleague offering a cigarette, passing a smoking zone) can create a craving for tobacco.

Thus, tobacco dependence is maintained not only by the positive reinforcement effects of nicotine and the conditioned stimuli associated with smoking, but also by the avoidance of the negative consequences of withdrawal.[1,6]

## Biological Theories

TD is mediated primarily by the actions of nicotine on brain nicotinic acetylcholine receptors (nAChRs). When a person smokes, the smoke particles containing nicotine enter the lungs, where nicotine is absorbed rapidly into circulation and moves quickly to the brain, as well as to the other parts of the body, where it binds to nAChRs. The nAChR complex is composed of five subunits and is found in both the peripheral and central nervous systems. The most abundant receptor subtypes in the brains of humans are α4 β2, α3 β4, and α7 (homomeric). The α4 β2 receptor subtype is predominant in the human brain and is the main receptor mediating nicotine dependence. In mice, knocking out the β2 subunit gene eliminates the behavioral effects of nicotine, including self-administration.[11–13] Reinserting the β2 subunit gene into the ventral tegmental area of the β2 knockout mouse restores behavioral responses to nicotine.[14] The α4 subunit is an important determinant of sensitivity to nicotine. Mutation of the α4subunit increases or decreases the nicotine-induced reward behaviors including tolerance to nicotine. The α3 β4 subunit and possibly the α7 homomeric receptor subtypes are believed to mediate the cardiovascular effects of nicotine.[15] The α7 subtype is also involved in rapid synaptic transmission and may play a role in learning and sensory gating, a component of conditioning.[16]

Stimulation of these receptors results in the release of a variety of brain neurotransmitters that produce arousal, mood modulation, and pleasure. Prolonged nicotine exposure results in neuroadaptation with desensitization and an increased number of nAChRs in the brain[6] (see Figure 3.3).

Our brains are wired to ensure that we will repeat life-sustaining activities by associating those activities with pleasure or reward.

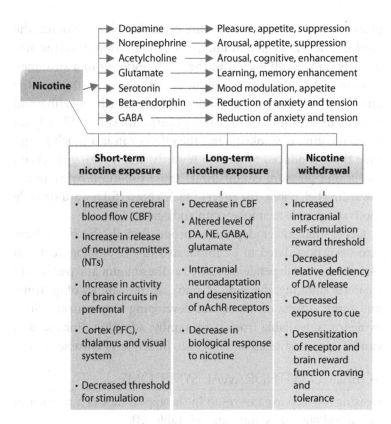

FIGURE 3.3   Brain changes in different phases of nicotine dependence. (From *Drugs, Brains, and Behavior: The Science of Addiction*.)

Whenever this reward circuit is activated, the brain notes that something important is happening that needs to be remembered, and teaches us to do it again and again. The "rewarding" effect of nicotine is attributed to its ability to activate the dopaminergic pathways projecting from the ventral tegmental area of the midbrain to the cerebral cortex and the limbic system.[1,5,6] The increase in dopamine in the nucleus accumbens is mediated by receptors in cell bodies in the ventral tegmental area (VTA). Food, for example, stimulates reward via the VTA which leads to dopamine overflow in the nucleus accumbens, which leads to pleasure. The "amount" of pleasure depends on how enjoyable the food is, and the degree of hunger. In comparison, nicotine acts directly on the cell bodies in the VTA resulting in a sustained response. When tobacco is used, it can release 2–10 times the amount of dopamine that natural rewards, such as eating and sex, do. In some individuals, this occurs almost immediately (as when nicotine is smoked), and the effects can last much longer than those produced by natural rewards. The resulting effects on the brain's pleasure circuit dwarf those produced by naturally rewarding behaviors. The effect of such a powerful reward strongly motivates people to smoke again and again.[4-6]

Genes that affect dopamine production in the brain have also been postulated to be implicated in the development and maintenance of dependence as well as the amount and patterns of cigarette smoking, duration of smoking, probability of quitting, and some aspects of the risk of developing lung cancer.[11] Such evidence is available from twin, family, adoption, linkage, and candidate gene studies, and has been linked to 14 chromosomes.

## TOBACCO WITHDRAWAL SYMPTOMS

Ceasing tobacco use can result in the appearance of a number of mood and physical symptoms (see Table 3.1).

TABLE 3.1    Tobacco Withdrawal—Mood and Physical Symptoms[17-20]

| Symptom/Physical Sign | Average Duration |
| --- | --- |
| Depressed mood | <4 weeks |
| Sleep disturbance | <2 weeks |
| Irritability | <4 weeks |
| Difficulty concentrating | <2 weeks |
| Restlessness | <4 weeks |
| Increased appetite and increased weight | >10 weeks |
| Constipation | > 4 weeks |
| Mouth ulcers | > 4 weeks |
| Light-headedness | <2 weeks |
| Urge to smoke | >10 weeks |

Many smokers suffer from withdrawal symptoms but to varying degrees of severity. However, tobacco withdrawal symptoms are mostly short-lived and people withdrawing from tobacco can be reassured that these should disappear within 4–6 weeks. Urges to smoke usually last longer, but do decrease in frequency and people can learn to manage these. Increased appetite can also last for longer than 6 weeks, and associated with this is weight gain (the average weight gained in the first year of abstinence is around 5 kg).

## BEHAVIORAL CONDITIONING OF THE NON-NICOTINE EFFECTS OF SMOKING

People habitually smoke cigarettes in specific situations, such as after a meal, with a cup of coffee or an alcoholic drink, or with friends who smoke. The association between smoking and these other events repeated many times causes the environmental situations to become powerful cues for the urge to smoke. Likewise, aspects of the drug-taking process, such as the manipulation of smoking materials, or the taste, smell, or feel of smoke in the throat, become associated with the pleasurable effects of smoking. Respiratory tract sensory cues associated with tobacco smoking represent a type of conditioned reinforcement that has been shown to play an important role in the regulation of smoke intake and the craving to smoke, as well as the rewarding effects of smoking.[21,22] Even unpleasant moods can become conditioned cues for smoking.[23] For example, a smoker may learn that not having a cigarette provokes irritability (a common symptom of tobacco withdrawal syndrome) and smoking a cigarette provides relief. After repeated experiences of this sort, a smoker may come to regard irritability from any source, such as stress or frustration, as a cue for smoking. Therefore, conditioned reinforcement could be the primary motivation to smoke during periods when desensitization prevents the reinforcing effects of nicotine obtained from smoking. This relationship is renewed on a cyclic basis. After a period of abstinence, when α4 β2 nAChRs are once again sensitive, the rewarding effects of smoking are reestablished and once again paired with the sensory stimuli of tobacco smoke, and the association of these two factors (stimuli and reward) is again strengthened. Conditioning is a major factor that causes relapse in drug use after a period of cessation, so it should be addressed as a component of counseling and behavioral therapy for TD. Also, such behavioral conditioning serves to maintain nicotine use during periods of desensitization of α4 β2 nAChRs, in which there is a loss or decrease in the biologic response to nicotine. Therefore, conditioned reinforcement could be the primary motivation to smoke during periods when desensitization prevents the reinforcing effects of nicotine obtained from smoking.[1,6,16]

To summarize, TD can best be understood and treated comprehensively using the biopsychosocial model[22] (see Figure 3.4) by taking factors related to all the aforementioned theories

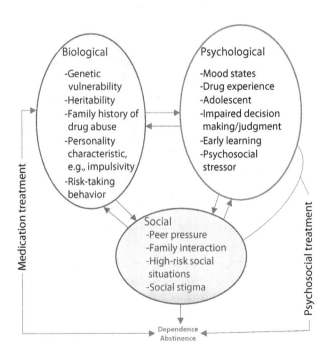

FIGURE 3.4   Biopsychosocial model of tobacco dependence.

into account, but in varied proportion from individual to individual.

## WHY SHOULD PRIMARY CARE PHYSICIANS KNOW ABOUT THEORIES OF TOBACCO DEPENDENCE?

Needless to say, in India, tobacco dependence (in various forms) is the most common form of substance dependence, has enormous physical health consequences, places a huge burden on the health care system, and is of enormous public health importance. More than 75% of smokers try to quit by themselves, but only 5%–10% quit permanently,[3,4] suggesting the need for professional help so as to increase the percentage of quitting. This quitting gap can possibly be bridged by primary care physicians and their work team in the primary health care system (as they are the first point of contact with people using tobacco products), which would be of immense help. The primary care physician and health workers can identify the people who are tobacco-dependent or those who are at risk of tobacco dependence. Then, they can help people understand why quitting can be difficult, and offer advice and support to help people cease tobacco use.

## CASE STUDY 2

### Hidden Igniter

Mr. Patel is a 32-year-old Indian lawyer, who is unmarried and lives with his parents and brother. He was admitted to a tertiary care general hospital for coughing up blood. On enquiry, Mr. Patel revealed that he started smoking cigarettes, occasionally, in the company of his friends when he was in standard 11. He lost his paternal grandmother, with whom he was very attached, in standard 12, and following this loss, he reported difficulty in concentration, was tense and feared that he would not be able to cope with the 12th board examination. As a remedy to overcome these problems, he started smoking more regularly. Mr. Patel also perceived that smoking helped him concentrate in his studies, and continued to smoke one packet of cigarettes a day. He scored well in the standard 12 examination, and subsequently joined a 5-year integrated law course.

Mr. Patel's mother is a reputed lawyer who is always busy with her clients, leaving little time for her son. His father works as a bank manager, was a smoker for 15 years and quit at 40. He also had a history of alcohol abuse. Mr. Patel was shy in nature, had very few friends, and was not comfortable in social situations. But, he wished he would have good social skills. At law school, he was not able to present seminars or presentations, or participate in group discussions unless he took some cigarettes. Subsequently, his cigarette consumption increased to two packets a day. At 22, he was diagnosed with chronic bronchitis, as a direct consequence of smoking, and his physician advised him to quit. He stopped smoking for 3 months, but when the final year law examinations approached, he relapsed to smoking again. Gradually, over the next couple of months, his pattern of smoking resumed to two packets a day. There would be frequent arguments with parents in relation to smoking, where they often called him "a person with weak willpower, a person with no determination." Over the next 10 years, Mr. Patel tried numerous times to quit, without success. Now in the hospital he was diagnosed as a case of stage I lung cancer, and also the reason for coughing up blood.

*Discussion of the case*: Mr. Patel is clearly tobacco-dependent with medical complications, including chronic bronchitis and lung cancer. He has risk factors as a result of a paternal history of drug abuse, he started using nicotine at an early age, he possesses poor social skills, and also possibly experienced a lack of parental supervision. Presumably, the availability of tobacco products was not an issue as he belonged to the upper class, and tobacco is not an illicit substance in India. He felt the short-term effects of nicotine as pleasurable, including better mood, feeling more alert with improved concentration, which helped him perform better. His learning and memory of the past drug experience, via conditioning, contributed to his relapse during the final law examination period.

**KEY MESSAGES**

- Tobacco dependence, as a brain disease, is best understood by the complex interaction between the genetic, biological, psychological, and social contributing factors
- Key to theories of dependence: Brain reward pathways using dopamine as a major mediating neurotransmitter, affect learning and conditioning
- Primary care physicians have an important role to play in:
  - The early identification of individuals with TD
  - Identification of risk factors, protective factors, and psychosocial issues, including the identification of cues and reinforcements in a given case
  - Communicating information about tobacco dependence that will help the tobacco user understand why they are dependent and what can be done to cease long-term tobacco use
  - Reassuring the client that effective treatment for tobacco withdrawal is available
  - Treating the coexisting medical condition and TD with equal emphasis
  - Taking effective practical measures to ensure the follow-up of such cases and intervening again if relapse occurs

## REFERENCES

1. Hughes JR. Nicotine-related disorders. In: Sadock BJ, Sadock VA, Pedro R (eds). *Kaplan & Sadock's Comprehensive Textbook of Psychiatry.* 9th ed. Philadelphia: Lippincott Williams & Wilkins; 2009, p.1353–1360.
2. The Science of Drug Abuse and Addiction. National Institute of Drug Abuse. http://www.drugabuse.gov/
3. Sadock BJ, Sadock VA, Pedro R. Tobacco related disorders. In: *Kaplan & Sadock's Synopsis of Psychiatry Behavioral Sciences/ Clinical Psychiatry.* 11th ed. New Delhi: Wolters Kluwer (India) Pvt Ltd; 2015, p. 680–685.
4. Sadock BJ, Sadock VA, Pedro R. Substance use and addictive disorders—Introduction and overview. In: *Kaplan & Sadock's Synopsis of Psychiatry Behavioral Sciences/Clinical Psychiatry.* 11th ed. New Delhi: Wolters Kluwer (India) Pvt Ltd; 2015, p. 616–624.

5. Drugs, Brains, and Behavior—The Science of Addiction. www.drugabuse.gov/publications/drugs-brains-behavior-science-addiction/drug-abuse-addiction.

6. Benowitz NL. Neurobiology of nicotine addiction: Implications for smoking cessation treatment. *Am J Med* 2008;121(4A):S3–S10.

7. Pianezza ML, Sellers EM, Tyndale RF. Nicotine metabolism defect reduces smoking. *Nature* 1998;393:750.

8. O'Brien CP. Research advances in the understanding and treatment of addiction. *Am J Addict* 2003;12(S2):36–47.

9. Le Foll B, Goldberg SR. Nicotine as a typical drug of abuse in experimental animals and humans. *Psychopharmacology* 2006;184: 367–81.

10. Padhy SK, Sarkar S, Khatana S. Media and mental Illness. *J Postgrad Med* 2014;60(2):163–170.

11. Loughlin JO, Paradis G, Kim W, DiFranza J, Meshefedjian G, McMillan-Davey E, Wong S, Hanley J, Tyndale R. Genetically decreased CYP2A6 and the risk of tobacco dependence: A prospective study of novice smokers. *TobControlv* 2004;13(4): 422–428.

12. Benowitz NL, Hukkanen J, Jacob P. Nicotine: Chemistry, metabolism, kinetics and biomarkers. *Handb Exp Pharmacol* 2009;(192):29–60.

13. Picciotto MR, Zoli M, Rimondini R et al. Acetylcholine receptors containing the 2 subunit are involved in the reinforcing properties of nicotine. *Nature* 1998;391:173–177.

14. Maskos U, Molles BE, Pons S et al. Nicotine reinforcement and cognition restored by targeted expression of nicotinic receptors. *Nature* 2005;436:103–107.

15. Aberger K, Chitravanshi VC, Sapru HN. Cardiovascular responses to microinjections of nicotine into the caudal ventrolateral medulla of the rat. *Brain Res* 2001;892:138–146.

16. Hajos M, Hurst RS, Hoffmann WE et al. The selective α7 nicotinic acetylcholine receptor agonist PNU-282987 [N-[(3R)-1-Azabicyclo [2.2.2]oct-3-yl]-4-chlorobenzamide hydrochloride] enhances GABAergic synaptic activity in brain slices and restores auditory gating deficits in anesthetized rats. *J PharmacolExpTher* 2005;312:1213–1222.

17. Hughes JR. Tobacco withdrawal in self-quitters. *J Consult Clin Psychol* 1992;60(5):689–697.

18. West R, Hajek P, Belcher M. Time course of cigarette withdrawal symptoms while using nicotine gum. *Psychopharmacology (Berl)* 1989;99(1):143–145.
19. Hajek P, Gillison F, McRobbie H. Stopping smoking can cause constipation. *Addiction* 2003;98(11):1563–1567.
20. McRobbie H, Hajek P, Gillison F. The relationship between smoking cessation and mouth ulcers. *Nicotine Tob Res* 2004;6(4):655–659.
21. Rose JE, Behm FM, Westman EC, Johnson M. Dissociating nicotine and nonnicotine components of cigarette smoking. *Pharmacol Biochem Behav* 2000;67:71–81.
22. Balfour DJ. The neurobiology of tobacco dependence: A preclinical perspective on the role of the dopamine projections to the nucleus. *Nicotine Tob Res.* 2004; 6:899–912.
23. Cloninger CR. The science of well-being: An integrated approach to mental health and its disorders. *World Psychiatry* 2006;5:71–76.

# CHAPTER 4

# Behavioral and Psychological Approaches for Tobacco Cessation

Sonali Jhanjee

## Objectives

The major objectives are to

- Learn evidence-based psychological and behavioral techniques to help people quit using tobacco
- Reflect on incorporating tobacco cessation counseling into routine medical consultations

## Skill Sets You Will Acquire

You will be able to conceptualize

- Knowledge about different psychological and behavioral techniques available for tobacco cessation

- Knowledge on brief interventions of tobacco cessation
- Awareness of common roadblocks in tobacco cessation
- Individual and group counseling techniques for tobacco cessation

## INTRODUCTION

Tobacco use is the leading cause of preventable death and kills nearly 6 million people worldwide each year.[1] Most tobacco users want to quit, but they are unable to do so as they are addicted to nicotine.[2] Relapse rates are staggeringly high and only about 5% of those who attempt to quit on their own achieve long-term abstinence.[3] Tobacco dependence is now conceptualized as a chronic relapsing illness that often requires repeated intervention and multiple attempts to quit. Tobacco dependence has both physiological and behavioral components. Stopping tobacco use causes distressing withdrawal symptoms, including craving, irritability, and insomnia—making it difficult to quit using tobacco. In addition to this, behavioral aspects may also make abstinence difficult. For example, relapses for tobacco use during quitting attempts may be triggered by environmental cues associated with smoking, such as seeing other people smoke, eating a meal, or drinking alcohol. These environmental stimuli or cues evoke cravings for the drug or drug-seeking behavior.[4,5] To treat tobacco users effectively, clinicians need to address both the physical and behavioral aspects of nicotine dependence. Established first-line treatments include pharmacological and behavioral interventions. This chapter discusses behavioral interventions for smoking cessation.

## CONCEPTUAL FRAMEWORK

Tobacco cessation interventions place central importance on the concept of motivation in the quitting process. The most widely used and popular theory of motivation is the Trans-Theoretical

Model (often referred to as the "Stages of Change Model"), which was proposed by Prochaska and DiClemente.[6] This model assumes that a smoker goes through a series of stages of behavior before quitting successfully, these stages include

- Pre-contemplation stage (not considering quitting)

- Contemplation stage (unsure)

- Preparation stage (ready)

- Action stage (reduced use or has quit for less than 6 months)

- Maintenance stage (those who have maintained the change for more than 6 months)

Relapse (resumption of old behaviors) can happen at any stage. Each stage may require a different kind of support, and the type of intervention should be tailored to the motivational stage. In the pre-contemplation/contemplation stage, use skills to help increase readiness for cessation, like motivational interviewing. Motivational Interviewing (MI) is a specific counseling strategy, which is intended to resolve ambivalence and increase a person's motivation for behavior change. MI strengthens the patient's "change talk" (e.g., reasons, ideas, needs for eliminating tobacco use) and "commitment language" (e.g., intentions to take action to change smoking behavior, such as not smoking in the home). Patients who have made plans to quit or who are in the process of quitting, are in the preparation/action stage and they may be given behavioral interventions and medicines to quit. Relapse prevention is important for patients in the maintenance stage.

Another recent theory describing smoking cessation is the "PRIME [Plans, Responses, Impulses, Motives, Evaluations] Theory of Motivation."[7] This theory proposes the initiation of quit attempts by offering help to all smokers without necessarily asking about their interest to quit. According to this theory, smokers' evaluative beliefs about smoking determine the decision for smoking cessation. The motivation, along with internal impulses to smoke and external triggers such as environmental cues, has an impact on their subsequent behavior.

On the one hand, the first (Trans-Theoretical Model) captures situations where a patient is able to stop smoking in a planned manner; on the other, the second (PRIME Model) is better at explaining spontaneous smoking cessation.

Accumulating evidence indicates that the likelihood of success in an attempt to quit is unrelated to the smoker's expressed interest in quitting.[8] This means that it is beneficial to encourage all smokers to consider quitting whenever the opportunity arises without the need to assess their readiness to quit.

## EVIDENCE-BASED APPROACHES

Behavioral approaches to tobacco cessation range in complexity from simple advice offered by a physician or other health care provider, to much more extensive therapy offered by counselors or specialized tobacco cessation services.

### Brief/Simple Advice/Minimal Clinical Intervention to Quit Tobacco

The simplest intervention for tobacco cessation is for a doctor to advise their patient to stop smoking. This may be done opportunistically during the course of a routine medical consultation. Clinicians can make a difference with even minimal (less than a minute) intervention. Brief advice to quit using tobacco can increase the chances of long-term abstinence by a further 2%–3%.[9] Whereas, the absolute effect of brief advice is relatively small, this intervention can have a considerable public health impact because of the large number of people who visit their doctors and the wide reach of primary care doctors.[5]

The 5A's approach for tobacco cessation (Figure 4.1) is one of the most commonly used methods for brief tobacco cessation interventions.[10]

The 5A's approach prompts health professionals to: "Ask" patients if they use tobacco; "Advise" on the importance of

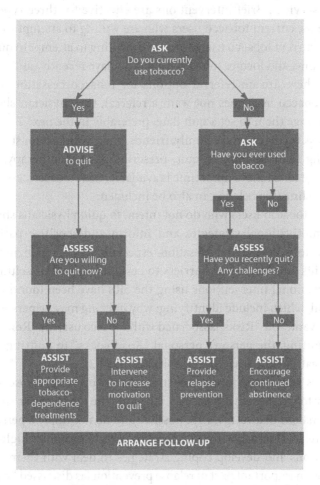

FIGURE 4.1 The 5A's Model. (From Fiore MC, Jaen CR, Baker TB et al. *Treating Tobacco Use and Dependence: 2008 Update. Quick Reference Guide for Clinicians.* USDHSS, 2009.)

quitting; "Assess" their willingness to *quit now*; offer "Assistance" in the form of pharmacotherapy and/or referral for behavioral support; and "Arrange" a follow-up appointment to check on their progress. This type of brief intervention is relatively inexpensive and cost-effective when integrated into existing primary health care services. Brief interventions are effective for three types of patients: current tobacco users who are willing to attempt to quit now, current tobacco users who are unwilling to attempt to quit at this time, and former tobacco users who have recently quit.

If there are no referral options for tobacco cessation, or if the tobacco user does not want a referral, the physician should encourage them to set a quit date, preferably in the next 2 weeks, and ask them to involve family, friends, and coworkers for support during their attempt to quit, prescribe pharmacotherapy, and arrange for a follow-up. If time is available, then tobacco cessation counseling (see below) can also be included.

For tobacco users who do not intend to quit, physicians should use motivational strategies and inform and sensitize patients about tobacco use and cessation, especially by personalizing the benefits and discussing barriers to cessation and their solutions. Motivational interventions using the 5R's have been found to be useful, which include identifying: why quitting may be personally "Relevant," the "Risks" associated with tobacco use, the "Rewards" of quitting, the person's personal "Roadblocks" to quitting, and "Repeating" the advice (see Tables 4.1 and 4.2).

It is important to discuss strategies to prevent relapse with every tobacco user who has recently quit. The tobacco user should understand that relapses are possible and do not imply a personal failure. It is important to teach tobacco users to recognize high-risk situations and develop coping strategies to deal with them. This forms an important part of relapse prevention (as discussed below).

### Self-Help Materials
Self-help information includes printed, written, or online materials that provide advice about ways to quit. They may also be

TABLE 4.1 The 5R's

| The 5R's | Details |
| --- | --- |
| Relevance | Help the individual identify why quitting tobacco is relevant to them. Information has the greatest impact when it is personalized in the context of a patient's disease status or risk, family, or social situation (e.g., having children in the home), other important patient characteristics (e.g., prior quitting experience, personal barriers to cessation). |
| Risks | Encourage the individual to verbalize possible negative outcomes of tobacco use like breathing difficulties, cancer, and heart disease. |
| Rewards | Help the individual identify the possible benefits of quitting such as improved health and financial well-being. |
| Roadblocks | Help the individual identify possible obstacles to quitting, including those from their past attempts to quit. These might include withdrawal symptoms, fear of failure, weight gain, lack of support, and depression (see Table 4.2). |
| Repetition | It might take more than just one brief intervention before a tobacco user is ready to quit. Use the 5A's at every visit! |

*Source:* Adapted from Fiore MC, Jaen CR, Baker TB, Bailey WC et al. *Treating Tobacco Use and Dependence: 2008 Update. Clinical Practice Guideline.* USDHSS , 2008.

TABLE 4.2 Common Roadblocks

| Belief | Possible Solution |
| --- | --- |
| "I can quit at any time/I'm not addicted." | The tobacco user should be asked about their past attempts to quit and success rates here. |
| Some users may consider asking for assistance as a sign of weakness. | They may be educated about unassisted quit rates of 3%–5%. |
| Smokeless tobacco use is harmless. Tobacco use is good for oral health. | Inform the user about the carcinogenic potential of smokeless tobacco. India has one of the highest rates of oral cancer in the world, which is related to tobacco chewing. |
| Tobacco use is good for oral health. | Tell them that tobacco use can actually cause great harm to oral health and in fact may cause premalignant and malignant lesions of the oral cavity! |
| Too addicted/too hard to quit. | Ask about previous attempts to quit. Discuss medications that can relieve withdrawal symptoms and counseling. |

available as audio recordings and videos/DVDs. Printed materials are most common and may range from a brief guide and tips to quit, to a structured manual with exercises to guide quit attempts. These self-help materials may be aimed at smokers in the general population (standard or generic), or individually tailored, which are based on the individual response of smokers at baseline, and their subsequent interactive feedback about their motivation, triggers for smoking, and coping skills. Standard, printed self-help materials increase quit rates compared to no intervention, but the effect is likely to be small. There is evidence that materials that are tailored for individual smokers are more effective than non-tailored materials, although the absolute size of the effect is still small (additional 1% of the unassisted quit rate of 2%–3%).[11] However, self-help materials have the advantage of being able to reach large numbers of people at a relatively low per-person cost and hence can be cost-effective.[12] The materials are appropriate in language, literacy level, and cultural approach. The increasing accessibility of the Internet should increase opportunities for individually tailored self-help therapies.

## Tobacco Cessation Counseling

Most behavioral interventions aim to develop motivation to resist the urge to use tobacco and develop a person's capacity to implement their plans to avoid tobacco use. These interventions are typically most helpful during the first few weeks of the quit attempt, where the strength of tobacco withdrawal syndrome is at its peak.[6] Tobacco cessation counseling can be delivered in different ways, including telephone, face-to-face, and web-based interventions.

Tobacco cessation programs often use a mix of cognitive and behavioral therapies. Cognitive therapy in smoking cessation aims to reframe a person's view of tobacco use and encourage patients to take a positive approach to cessation by employing distraction techniques and relaxation methods. Behavioral therapy aims to help smokers recognize the stimuli associated with the act of smoking and avoid such triggers by modifying their behavior, and also help patients address the consequences of tobacco withdrawal, such as craving.[13]

Research has elucidated a number of evidence-based behavior change techniques that are associated with a high likelihood of tobacco cessation. Tobacco cessation counselors should be competent in these techniques (see the box below). More practical advice is provided in the section below on face-to-face counseling.

---

**COMPETENCIES REQUIRED TO DELIVER BEHAVIORAL SUPPORT FOR STOPPING SMOKING**

**This research was undertaken in the UK where smoking is the predominant form of tobacco use.[14,15]**

For individual treatment, required competencies include:

- Developing rapport and eliciting client views
- Assessing current and past smoking behavior, including past quit attempts
- Assessing the person's current readiness and ability to stop
- Facilitating goal setting and action planning (including the development of a treatment plan)
- Providing advice on stop-smoking medications
- Prompting and gaining commitment from the client there and then
- Using a carbon monoxide monitor to measure carbon monoxide levels during each session (only applies to face-to-face services and the use of smoked tobacco)
- Providing information on withdrawal symptoms
- Providing advice on changing routines, facilitating the identification of barriers to stopping, and to maintaining cessation, and problem solving
- Providing rewards/praise for stopping smoking
- Asking about the person's experience with stop-smoking medicines (current or previous); this includes monitoring for adverse effects

- Facilitating coping and identifying relapse prevention strategies
- Providing options for additional and later support
- Assisting the client with strengthening their new ex-smoker identity
- Providing appropriate written materials, as well as information on the consequences of smoking and stopping smoking

Group-based treatment requires the competencies for individual treatment (identified above), plus encouraging:

- Group discussions
- Group tasks that promote group interaction or bonding
- Mutual support

## Telephone Counseling and Quitlines

Telephone counseling is defined as the provision of telephone calls to aid in smoking cessation. Quitlines are a low-cost, popular, and easily accessible intervention that can reach a large number of smokers and can be available for extended hours. They provide confidential and anonymous support to smokers wanting to quit. Telephone helplines use two main approaches: reactive, in which smokers can simply telephone the line, and proactive, in which counselors ring callers back and give ongoing telephone support. Telephone counseling may be provided in addition to individual counseling, or substitute for individual counseling as an adjunct to self-help interventions or pharmacotherapy. The effectiveness and cost-effectiveness of proactive telephone counseling for smoking cessation is now widely recognized.[16] There is some evidence of a dose response; one or two brief calls are less likely to provide a measurable benefit. Three or more calls increase the chances of quitting compared to minimal intervention such as providing standard self-help materials, or brief advice, or compared to pharmacotherapy alone.[17] Telephone smoking cessation counseling has been shown to be effective, and as a result has subsequently been integrated as a routine health care provision in many countries.

## Text Messages for Smoking Cessation

There is good evidence showing that text messages, delivered through mobile phones, are effective in helping people stop smoking in the long term.[18] This type of intervention is also one of the most affordable interventions available to all countries.

## Newer Technology-Based Interventions

Internet (web-based) interventions are delivered through the use of a computer. The tobacco user may navigate within a specific website to access general treatment or interact with a program that delivers a tailored intervention. Results suggest that some Internet-based interventions can assist with smoking cessation, especially if the information is appropriately tailored to the users.[19] However, trials have not shown consistent effects and more evidence is needed to determine if this can help people stop smoking. Given their broad reach and low costs, technology-based interventions remain a highly promising delivery system for reducing tobacco dependence.

## Face-to-Face Counseling (Individual and Group Based)

Behavioral support, with multiple sessions of individual or group counseling, assists smoking cessation. Individual counseling involves scheduled face-to-face appointments with a trained smoking cessation counselor. Individual counseling has been found to be effective as demonstrated by a systematic review which found that the relative risk (RR) for smoking cessation at long-term follow-up was 1.39, 95% confidence interval (CI) 1.24–1.57.[15] Multiple and longer sessions appear to be more effective and four or more sessions that are 10 minutes or more in length appear to be especially effective in increasing abstinence rates.[10]

Group counseling is offered to small groups (typically 10–20 people) of clients, and in this setting, clients can share problems and derive support from one another. The chances of quitting smoking are approximately doubled. Groups are usually led by trained facilitators with skills while conducting group-based treatment.[10]

Both individual and group therapy have been shown to improve quit rates beyond those seen with self-help materials alone and other less intensive interventions. There appears to be no difference between individual and group therapy in terms of quit rates.[10]

## Practical Counseling Techniques (Adapted from Fiore et al., 2008)[10]

The following techniques can be helpful when treating tobacco use and dependence in both individual and group counseling.[14]

### Provide Basic Information

Provide basic information about tobacco use and successful quitting, including:

- The addictive nature of smoking or smokeless tobacco use
- Any use (e.g., a single smoke/chew) increases the likelihood of a full relapse
- Withdrawal typically peaks within 1–3 weeks after quitting

### Learning to Cope with Urges/Cravings to Use Tobacco

Cravings or the urge to use tobacco is experienced by most tobacco users when they quit. Cravings begin within hours after stopping, and typically peak within the first 1–2 weeks of the attempt to quit. The craving for tobacco can last long term, but as the days pass, the cravings become further and further apart. Reassure users that craving is common but will ease over time. Suggesting simple techniques, such as the "Five D's," may be helpful in managing cravings, these include:

- *Delay* until the urge passes—usually within minutes: Remind yourself that cravings are temporary. The urge will pass in a few minutes. Don't give in.
- *Distract* yourself: Take a bath or go for a walk.
- *Drink* water to fight off cravings.

- *Deep* breaths—Relax! Close your eyes and take 10 slow, deep breaths.

- *Discuss* your feelings with someone close to you.

## Identify Triggers and Recognize Danger (High-Risk) Situations

The patient should make a personal list or be aware of "triggers". Triggers are situations, places, or feelings that make that person more likely to use tobacco. Being aware of these can help to avoid them or at least be ready for them. These can be external situations (seeing others smoking or chewing tobacco; passing by a shop selling tobacco; a social function where many persons are using tobacco; contact with tobacco accessories such as matchboxes or lighters, seeing an empty pouch or sachet on the road) or internal situations (feeling lonely, sad, anxious, irritated, dull, or angry) which bring on the urge or craving. Identify events, internal states, or activities that increase the risk of tobacco use or relapse, for example,

- Negative mood
- Being around other smokers or smokeless tobacco users
- Drinking alcohol
- Experiencing urges/cravings
- Being under time pressure
- Develop coping skills

Identify and practice coping or problem-solving skills. These skills are intended to cope with danger situations (high-risk situations) to avoid relapse (relapse prevention).

Learn to anticipate: for example, facing the morning. When you wake up, think of alternatives to using tobacco. Be sure that there are no cigarettes, bidis, packets are available. Begin each day with a pre-planned activity that will keep you busy for an hour or more.

Avoid temptation: Learn the 4A's

- *Avoid*: Certain people and places can tempt you to use tobacco. Avoid others while they're using tobacco. Refuse offers of tobacco.

- *Alter*:

  - Switch to water instead of alcohol or tea

  - Take a different route to school or work

  - Take a walk when you feel the need to take a smoke/smokeless tobacco break

- *Alternatives*: For smokeless tobacco users there is often a stronger need to have something in the mouth (oral substitute) to take the place of the chew or pouch. Hence, use oral substitutes such as gum, cloves, or saunf.

- *Activities*: Exercise or "engage in" hobbies that keep your hands busy, which can help can help distract.

### Other

The patient may complain of other problems such as difficulty in concentration, irritability, and insomnia. However, the patient may be counseled that these problems are temporary and will likely resolve within a month. Relaxation techniques can also be taught.

### Provision for Social Support

*Intra-treatment social support*: Provide a supportive clinical environment while encouraging the patient with his or her quit attempt. The team at the primary care facility may always indicate their support, advice, and availability if the patient is faced with problems during a quit attempt.

*Extra-treatment social support:* Help your patients develop social support for the attempt to quit by involving family members. It is important to tell family members that quitting tobacco is difficult for the patient; it is not just a matter of willpower.

## Other Behavioral Techniques

Over time, many behavioral techniques have been tried for tobacco cessation. But none of them have a strong evidence base. Acupuncture and hypnotherapy have not been shown to be effective for tobacco cessation. Aversion therapy pairs the pleasurable stimulus of smoking a cigarette with some unpleasant stimulus. The objective is to extinguish the urge to smoke. Aversive smoking involves rapid smoking, where the patient smokes intensively, often to the point of discomfort, nausea, or vomiting. However, the effectiveness of aversive smoking has not been established. At present it is not recommended and appears not to be widely acceptable.[10]

## Combined Interventions

Quit rates are the highest when counseling is combined with pharmacotherapy. As a general rule, the more intensive the intervention, the better is the outcome.

## CONCLUSION

A wealth of evidence now indicates that behavioral interventions for tobacco cessation are effective. However, behavioral techniques still remain underutilized. Every health care provider must use the contact as an opportunity for assessing tobacco use behavior and promoting behavior change by providing treatment. It is important to incorporate these techniques in routine clinical practice in all health care settings. Integrating tobacco cessation services in primary care is essential to counter the magnitude of tobacco use in India.

## CASE STUDIES 3 AND 4

### Case 3

Ramesh, a 39-year-old IT professional, has been smoking since the age of 23 years. He smokes 15–20 cigarettes per day. He has his first smoke within 15 minutes after waking up. He believes that he is addicted to smoking. He is however willing to quit but is scared of the withdrawal symptoms associated with it. Ramesh visits his physician asking for help.

What should the physician do?

### Case 4

Satish, a 57-year-old man visits a general physician to talk about his smoking habit but has been forced to do so by his wife, who wants him to quit.

*Doc:* So you have been forced to see me by your wife. Why did she want you to do so?

*Satish:* She has a problem with me smoking and it's been almost 6 months that she has been constantly complaining about me smoking.

*Doc:* Ok. Why do you think she is doing that?

*Satish:* Well, she is worried about my health and I get that, but I have been smoking all my life. My father is 85 and he smokes too. I don't think I am ready to quit. I don't think I can.

*Doc:* How do you think your smoking is affecting your life?

*Satish:* Well for starters, it has been causing problems between me and my wife. Even my kids have ganged up against me, and want me to quit. I don't know how I can manage to do that. I don't even smoke inside the house. I don't know what to do.

*Doc:* It seems your family wants you to quit, but you are unsure.

*Satish:* Yes. But I don't want my smoking to affect my family life.

*Doc:* Ok, that is a good sign. You don't have to quit all at once. You can slowly quit smoking. We can work on a plan to do so.

*Satish:* Oh, I can slowly quit? That is nice. I wish my wife was with me now, because it is like she wants me to quit immediately. May I bring her with me the next time I visit?

*Doc:* Sure you can. We can schedule another appointment and should start your quitting plan.

**KEY MESSAGES**

- It is essential to screen for and identify tobacco use consistently in all health care settings
- It is important that physicians ask about tobacco use status for all their patients, advise *all* tobacco users to stop on a regular basis and offer them assistance to quit
- All doctors and other health professionals should provide brief advice as a low intensity but routine intervention to all tobacco users

## REFERENCES

1. *WHO report on the global tobacco epidemic, 2009: Implementing smoke-free environments.* Geneva: World Health Organization, 2009. http://www.who.int/tobacco/mpower/2009/en/index.html, accessed August 27, 2013.
2. 2. Royal College of Physicians. *Nicotine addiction in Britain. A report of the Tobacco Advisory Group of the Royal College of Physicians.* London: Royal College of Physicians, 2000. Available at https://www.rcplondon.ac.uk/publications/nicotine-addiction-britain. Accessed on January 4, 2015.
3. Hughes JR, Keely J, Naud S. Shape of the relapse curve and long-term abstinence among untreated smokers. *Addiction* 2004;99(1): 29–38.
4. Cosci F, Pistelli F, Lazzarini N, Carrozzi L. Nicotine dependence and psychological distress: Outcomes and clinical implications in smoking cessation. *Psychol Res Behav Manage* 2011;4:119–28.
5. Aveyard P, Raw M. Improving smoking cessation approaches at the individual level. *Tob Control* 2012 Mar;21(2):252–7. DOI: 10.1136/tobaccocontrol-2011-0503486.
6. Prochaska JO, DiClemente CC. Stages and processes of self-change of smoking: Toward an integrative model of change. *J Consult Clin Psychol* 1983;51(3):390–5.

7. West R. *Theory of Addiction*. Oxford: Blackwell, 2006.
8. West R, Sohal T. "Catastrophic" pathways to smoking cessation: Findings from national survey. *BMJ* 2006;332:458–60.
9. Stead LF, Buitrago D, Preciado N, Sanchez G, Hartmann-Boyce J, Lancaster T. Physician advice for smoking cessation. *Cochrane Database Syst Rev* 2013;(5):CD000165. DOI: 10.1002/14651858. CD000165.pub4
10. Fiore MC, Jaen CR, Baker TB, Bailey WC et al. for the Guideline Panel. *Treating Tobacco Use and Dependence: 2008 Update. Clinical Practice Guideline*. Rockville, MD: U.S. Department of Health and Human Services. Public Health Service, May 2008. Available at www.surgeongeneral.gov/tobacco/treating_tobacco_use08.pdf.
11. Hartmann-Boyce J, Lancaster T, Stead LF. Print-based self-help interventions for smoking cessation. *Cochrane Database Syst Rev* 2014;(6):CD001118. DOI: 10.1002/14651858.CD001118.pub3.
12. Lancaster T, Stead LF. Self-help interventions for smoking cessation. In: *Cochrane Collaboration. Cochrane Library*. Issue 3. Oxford: Update Software, 2000.
13. Schroeder SA. What to do with a patient who smokes. *JAMA* 2005;294:482–7.
14. Michie S, Churchill S, West R. Identifying evidence-based competences required to deliver behavioral support for smoking cessation. *Ann Behav Med* 2011;41(1):59–70.
15. Michie S, Hyder N, Walia A et al. Development of a taxonomy of behavior change techniques used in individual behavioral support for smoking cessation. *Addict Behav* 2011;36(4):315–19.
16. Lancaster T, Stead LF. Individual behavioural counselling for smoking cessation. *Cochrane Database Syst Rev* 2005;(2):CD001292. DOI: 10.1002/14651858. CD001292.pub2.
17. Stead LF, Hartmann-Boyce J, Perera R, Lancaster T. Telephone counselling for smoking cessation. *Cochrane Database Syst Rev* 2013;(8):CD002850. DOI: 10.1002/14651858. CD002850.pub3.
18. Whittaker R, McRobbie H, Bullen C, Borland R, Rodgers A, Gu Y. Mobile phone-based interventions for smoking cessation. *Cochrane Database Syst Rev* 2012 Nov 14;11:CD006611. DOI: 10.1002/14651858. CD006611.pub3.
19. Civljak M, Sheikh A, Stead LF, Car J. Internet-based interventions for smoking cessation. *Cochrane Database Syst Rev* 2010;(9):CD007078. DOI: 10.1002/14651858. CD007078.pub3.
20. Fiore MC, Jaen CR, Baker TB et al. *Treating Tobacco Use and Dependence: 2008 Update. Quick Reference Guide for Clinicians*. Rockville, MD: U.S. Department of Health and Human Services. Public Health Service, April 2009.

# CHAPTER 5

# Pharmacological Approaches for Tobacco Cessation

Binod Kumar Patro and Suravi Patra

**Objectives**

The major objectives are to

- Provide an overview of the use of pharmacotherapy in addition to counseling for tobacco cessation

- Provide an understanding of the selection of medication depending on a patient's level of tobacco use, personal preference, and physical comorbidities

- Describe an empathic and personalized treatment plan with regular follow-up

**Skill Sets You Will Acquire**

You will be able to conceptualize

- Knowledge about different pharmacological agents available for tobacco cessation
- Selection of pharmacological agents as per the level of dependence and associated conditions
- Monitoring the response to pharmacotherapy
- Tobacco cessation pharmacotherapy in special situations

## INTRODUCTION

Tobacco cessation is considered to be the gold standard of all preventive interventions as beneficial effects start immediately after the cessation of tobacco use.[1,2] Despite the evidence of the effectiveness of tobacco cessation interventions, they remain underutilized by physicians owing to a host of factors which include time constraints, clinician's own beliefs about lack of efficacy of interventions, and lack of knowledge and skills.[3]

Pharmacotherapy can play an important role in helping people cease tobacco use, and will roughly double the chances of long-term abstinence compared to placebo. The evidence presented in this chapter comes from studies that helped people stop smoking tobacco. Trials of some smoking cessation medicines have been conducted in people who use oral tobacco, but the results are mixed and further data are required. As noted in the previous chapter, a combination of behavioral support and pharmacotherapy results in the greatest chances of quitting.

Pharmacological agents used in smoking cessation are broadly classified into two groups.

1. *First-line agents*:

   - Nicotine replacement therapy (NRT)
   - Bupropion hydrochloride
   - Varenicline tartarate

2. *Second-line agents*:

- Nortriptyline
- Clonidine

Pharmacotherapy should be recommended to all smokers. The choice of medication will depend on a number of patient-related factors (see Table 5.1).

## FIRST-LINE AGENTS

### Nicotine Replacement Therapy

Nicotine has 100% bioavailability when smoked. Within seconds of inhalation, nicotine causes the release of neurotransmitters like dopamine that produces immediate feelings of relaxation and relieves withdrawal symptoms. Abstinence from tobacco product use reduces blood nicotine levels and triggers withdrawal symptoms (see Chapter 3).[5] These peak 48 hours after quitting, mostly subside by the end of the second week, and rarely last beyond a month.

Nicotine replacement therapy (NRT) was the first proven effective agent for the treatment of tobacco dependence. NRT alleviates tobacco withdrawal symptoms and craving experienced by tobacco users, making quitting a little easier.[6] There are various

TABLE 5.1   Factors Governing Medications of Choice[4]

| Belief | Possible Solution |
|---|---|
| Existing scientific evidence | Primary concern in deciding the medication on the basis of evidence of efficacy and safety. |
| Patient's preference | Based on patient's expectation and level of comfort with the medication. |
| Patient's experience | Patient's prior experience with the medication in terms of perceived success in an attempt to quit needs to be taken into account. |
| Comorbidities | For example, the presence of a seizure disorder proscribes against (denounces) the prescription of bupropion. |
| Patient needs | Based on patient's severity, extent, situations, and time of cravings, high-risk situations, and barriers. |

types of NRT such as patch, gum, tablet, lozenge, spray, and so on. In India nicotine gum and nicotine patch are available in different doses (Table 5.2).

### Principles of NRT Use[7]

1. *Dosage as per need*: NRT dose should be chosen depending on the amount of tobacco use. Level of dependence should be assessed by using the Fagerström test for nicotine dependence. Need for smoking within the first hour of getting up in the morning and 10 or more cigarettes smoked per day indicate high dependence. Nicotine gum of 4 mg and/or a nicotine patch of 21 mg should be prescribed in these cases, while lower doses should be used in cases of low dependence. The dose should be sufficient to prevent cravings. The presence of cravings is a pointer toward the inadequate dose of NRT.

2. Monitor for symptoms like nausea, headache, and palpitations that might be due to overdose, and reduce the dose of NRT.

3. Advise the patient to continue the use of NRT, even if they lapse. As this can prevent progression of lapse to relapse.

4. The type of NRT should be chosen on the basis of the patient's level of dependence, preference, and coexisting medical conditions. For example, in patients with allergy to sticking plaster, a patch might not be suitable, while those who cannot chew gum should not be prescribed with gum.

### Nicotine Gum

It is available in 2 mg or 4 mg formulations. A higher dose should be used in more highly dependent smokers.

The patient should be taught the "bite and park method" when using nicotine gum. They should bite the gum several times until a peppery taste or a tingling sensation appears. They should then

TABLE 5.2 Medications for Tobacco Cessation

| | Nicotine Replacement Therapy | Bupropion Hydrochloride | Varenicline Tartrate |
|---|---|---|---|
| Trade name and dose availability | Nicorette 2 mg, 4 mg<br>Nulife 2 mg, 4 mg<br>Nicotex 2 mg, 4 mg<br>Kwiknil 2 mg, 4 mg<br>Nicotine patch—2 Baconil 7 mg, 14 mg, and 21 mg | Bupron SR 150 mg<br>Zyban 150 mg<br>Bupep 150 mg | Champix 0.5 mg, 1 mg |
| Starting | On quit day | 1–2 weeks before quit date | 1–2 weeks before quit date |
| Dose regimen | *High dependence:* 4 mg every<br>1. 2 hours for 6 weeks, then every<br>2. 4 hours for 3 weeks, then every 4–8 hours for 3 weeks<br><br>*Low dependence:* 2 mg every 1–2 hours for 6 weeks, then every 2–4 hours for 3 weeks and then, every 4–8 hours for 3 weeks<br><br>*Use of tobacco within less than 30 minutes of morning awakening or greater than or equal to 20 cigarettes per day. If either of these criteria is not met, then the patient has low dependence[7]*<br><br>No more than 24 pieces in 24 hours<br><br>**Dosage regimen for nicotine patches**<br><br>**>10 cigarettes per day regimen**<br>1–6 weeks: 21 mg patch once daily<br>7–8 weeks: 14 mg patch once daily<br>9–10 weeks: 7 mg patch once daily<br><br>**<10 cigarettes per day regimen**<br>1–6 weeks: 14 mg patch once daily<br>7–8 weeks: 7 mg patch once daily | Bupron SR 150 mg OD for 3 days then 150 mg BD<br>Continue treatment for 7–12 weeks if there are signs of progress | 0.5 mg OD for 1–3 days,<br>then 0.5 mg BD for 4 days,<br>then 1 mg BD for 12 weeks |

(Continued)

TABLE 5.2 (*Continued*)  Medications for Tobacco Cessation

| | Nicotine Replacement Therapy | Bupropion Hydrochloride | Varenicline Tartrate |
|---|---|---|---|
| Adverse effects | Local mouth irritation<br>Jaw pain<br>Hiccups<br>Dyspepsia<br>Rhinitis<br>Nausea<br>Flatulence | Agitation<br>Anxiety<br>Dizziness<br>Headache<br>Insomnia<br>Constipation<br>Dry mouth<br>Nausea<br>Hypersensitivity reactions<br>Seizures (risk 1 in 1000) | Nausea<br>Headache<br>Dizziness<br>Somnolence<br>Fatigue<br>Sleep disturbances<br>Increased appetite and GI disturbances including vomiting, constipation, and flatulence<br>Depressed mood<br>Agitation |
| Cautions while prescribing | Hypersensitivity<br>Pregnancy | History of hypertension<br>Liver failure<br>Kidney failure | Serious neuropsychiatric disorders<br>History of suicidal, homicidal, or assaultive behavior within past 12 weeks<br>Untreated or unstable mental disorders<br>Severe renal impairment |

(*Continued*)

TABLE 5.2 (*Continued*) Medications for Tobacco Cessation

| | Nicotine Replacement Therapy | Bupropion Hydrochloride | Varenicline Tartrate |
|---|---|---|---|
| Contra-indication | Not to be sold to those below 18 years age<br>TMJ syndrome (for gum) | History of seizures<br>Predisposition to seizures (severe head trauma, CNS tumor)<br>Abrupt withdrawal from heavy alcohol or sedative use<br>Within 14 days of use of MAO inhibitors<br>Eating disorders (bulimia/anorexia nervosa)<br>Hypersensitivity<br>Pregnancy | |
| Advise | Check the patient technique for using the gum<br>Can be used in combination for better results | Use with caution in patients with liver/renal failure<br>Avoid in patients on MAO inhibitors<br>Monitor for neuropsychiatric signs and symptoms during use | Can be used as first-line therapy if patient prefers and does not have any contraindications<br>Ask about psychiatric history prior to prescribing and neuropsychiatric signs and symptoms during use |

*Note:* The bold text signifies the dependence on tobacco use, whereas the bold italic text is the criteria for the same.

stop chewing and park the gum in the inside of their cheek. Nicotine will be absorbed here. On disappearance of the tingling sensation and peppery taste, they should bite the gum again and again park the gum near their cheek. This process should be repeated. The patient should not continuously chew the gum as they may experience heartburn or stomach upset. The gum should be changed once it stops producing the tingling sensation or peppery taste.

Patients should be advised not to eat or drink for 15 minutes before, during, and after using gum. Nicotine gum contains sodium carbonate/bicarbonate, which increases the salivary pH to enhance nicotine absorption across the buccal mucosa, but acidic beverages like tea, coffee, juice inhibit nicotine absorption and should be avoided within 15 minutes of use.

Nicotine plasma levels peak approximately 30 minutes after chewing a piece of gum and slowly decline over 2–3 hours, and provides plasma concentration of 30%–64% of pre-cessation levels. Patients should be advised to use the gum regularly, every hour, for example.

### Nicotine Patches

Nicotine patches come in two different preparations—a 16-hour and a 24-hour patches. There is no difference in efficacy between these two types and so a choice can be made on the basis of availability and patient preference. Each preparation comes in three different strengths (16 hour: 25, 15, and 10 mg; 24 hour: 21, 14, and 7 mg). In general, smokers can start on the high-strength patch and use this for at least 8 weeks. The medium- and low-dose patches can be used for weaning, although this is not strictly necessary. For less-dependent smokers, starting on the medium strength patches may be more appropriate.

Patches should be applied to a clean, dry, and hairless area of skin. They should be kept in place for the recommended duration (16 or 24 hours) and then removed and disposed of. It is common to experience a little itching and redness under the patch.

*Combination Treatment*
Combination NRT has higher abstinence rates with no additional safety concerns. A higher dose of NRT is more effective than a lower dose of NRT in patients with higher severity of dependence. NRT is decided on the basis of patient preference. In addition, combination treatment is beneficial in cases of a failed attempt with monotherapy, breakthrough cravings, multiple failed attempts, or persisting nicotine withdrawal.[4]

*Bidi Smokers*
A bidi stick contains approximately 80% of nicotine contained in a manufactured cigarette, so the same dosage may also be applicable for bidi users.[8]

## Bupropion Hydrochloride

Bupropion hydrochloride sustained-release tablet is licensed as a non-nicotine tobacco cessation drug. Bupropion blocks dopamine–norepinephrine reuptake in the mesolimbic system and nucleus accumbens and also has a nicotine receptor blocking activity.[9] Its antismoking effect is independent of its antidepressant effect, and acts primarily to decrease nicotine withdrawal symptoms and craving.[10] Bupropion is as effective as NRT but less effective than varenicline. Bupropion should be started at least 1 week before the patient's quit date. For the first 3 days, one tablet daily should be taken, on the 4th day, one tablet twice daily should be taken to be continued for at least 7 weeks. In case of no improvement in abstinence, it should be withdrawn. For more information, refer to Table 5.2.

*Special Precautions*
- Neuropsychiatric symptoms should be monitored in patients prescribed with bupropion and patients should be informed about this prior to initiating the dose. These symptoms include depressed mood, suicidality, changes in behavior, hostility, agitation, and attempted suicide.

- These symptoms might appear in patients without preexisting psychiatric illness, and might worsen in those with preexisting psychiatric treatment.

- These symptoms should be monitored in patients even after they discontinue bupropion and be adequately managed.

### Drug Interactions

There are a number of interactions with bupropion that must be checked before prescribing. For example, carbamazepine may increase the metabolism of bupropion and reduce its efficacy.[11] Caution is needed when prescribing bupropion with drugs that lower seizure threshold like neuroleptics, lithium, tricyclic antidepressants, and alcohol. When used with ritonavir, a dose-dependent reduction in bupropion levels occurs.

### Varenicline Tartrate

Varenicline tartrate is a partial agonist of $\alpha 4\beta 2$-nicotinic acetylcholine receptor. Its action on nAChRs gives rise to dopamine release in the nucleus accumbens, thereby alleviating tobacco withdrawal. It also exerts an antagonistic effect on the $\alpha 4\beta 2$ receptor and so blocks nicotine induced dopaminergic activation and so reduces reward from smoking.[12] There are relatively few contraindications (pregnant and breastfeeding women, age <18 years), and no clinical relevant drug interactions. The most common side effects are nausea and gastrointestinal symptoms. Post-marketing surveillance found that some people reported severe neuropsychiatric adverse events and although no causality has been established, patients should be advised about the occurrence of such symptoms and followed up.

## SECOND-LINE AGENTS[13]

### Clonidine

It is a centrally acting $\alpha 2$ adrenergic agonist that depresses the sympathetic nervous system. Preliminary data show its efficacy in tobacco cessation but side effects limit its use.

TABLE 5.3   Effectiveness of Different Pharmacological Agents[14]

| Intervention | Comparator | Odds Ratio/Relative Risk (95% CI) |
| --- | --- | --- |
| Nicotine replacement therapy | Placebo | 1.84 (1.71–1.99) |
| Bupropion hydrochloride | Placebo | 1.80 (1.60–2.06) |
| Varenicline tartrate | Placebo | 2.88 (2.40–3.47) |
| Nortriptyline | Placebo | 2.03 (1.48–2.78) |
| Clonidine | Placebo | 1.63 (1.22–2.18) |

## Nortriptyline

It is a tricyclic antidepressant which blocks the reuptake of norepinephrine and serotonin. Its efficacy in tobacco cessation is almost similar to that of varenicline (Table 5.3).

## SPECIAL POPULATIONS[13]

### Psychiatric Comorbidity

Patients with psychiatric disorders like schizophrenia, bipolar disorder, and depressive disorders have a higher prevalence of tobacco dependence as compared to the general population. These patients can be given any medication effective for tobacco cessation keeping the contraindication in view.

### Pregnancy

Smoking during pregnancy increases the risk of both maternal and fetal morbidity. Nicotine use in pregnancy is not completely safe; however, NRT is considered safer than continued smoking as it only provides nicotine without the many other toxicants in tobacco smoke. The nicotine levels in blood when using NRT are also lower than those seen when smoking. Pregnant women can choose a form of NRT; however, if a patch is used, it should be removed before bedtime. Bupropion and varenicline are contraindicated in pregnancy.

### Adolescents

NRT can be considered in this population, but the level of tobacco dependence and patient preference has to be taken into consideration when deciding the treatment plan.

## CASE STUDY 5

A case study of the participants in the form of medical vignettes is essential to understand the context practically, if possible.

Vignesh, a 54-year-old banker, went to his primary care doctor with cough and chest pain that lasted for 15 days. On enquiry, he admitted smoking cigarettes since age 18 with current use of 10–12 cigarettes per day. His severity was assessed to be of low dependency on the basis of the Fagerström test score. On physical examination, the doctor recommended some tests and advised him to stop smoking stating the risk of respiratory and cardiac diseases. Vignesh further reported being pestered by his wife and teenage daughter to quit smoking, which he had not been able to do owing to his incapability to manage his cravings. The doctor provided him assistance by asking him to set a quit date and to start nicotine gum of 2 mg every 1–2 hours. He further arranged for a follow-up visit after 1 week to monitor his progress.

**KEY MESSAGES**

- Use of smoking cessation medicines increases long-term quit rates
- Best results are achieved when pharmacotherapy is used in combination with behavioral support
- NRT is available as an over-the-counter product in India
- Bupropion SR and varenicline are drugs available through prescription only
- Specific scientific evidence for use of pharmacotherapy among non-cigarette users in the Indian context is lacking; nevertheless, as nicotine is the addictive content in all non-cigarette tobacco products, NRT can be prescribed

## REFERENCES

1. Eddy DM. David Eddy ranks the tests. *Harv Health Lett* 1992;17(suppl):10–11.
2. Pimple S, Pednekar M, Mazumdar P, Goswami S, Shastri S. Predictors of quitting tobacco—Results of a worksite tobacco

cessation service program among factory workers in Mumbai, India. *Asian Pac J Cancer Prev* 2012;13(2):533–8.

3. Greden JF, Pomerleau O. Caffeine-related disorders and nicotine-related disorders. In: Kaplan HI, Sadock BJ, Cancro R (eds). *Comprehensive Textbook of Psychiatry.* 6th ed. Baltimore: Williams & Wilkins; 1995, p. 806–11.

4. Bader P, McDonald P, Selby P. An algorithm for tailoring pharmacotherapy for smoking cessation: Results from a Delphi panel of international experts. *Tob Control* 2009;18:34–42.

5. McLaughlin I, Dani JA, De Biasi M. Nicotine withdrawal. *Curr Top Behav Neurosci.* 2015;24:99–123.

6. Benowitz NL. Clinical pharmacology of nicotine: Implications for understanding, preventing, and treating tobacco addiction. *Clin Pharmacol Ther* 2008;83(4):531–41.

7. Fiore MC, Jaén CR, Baker TB, Bailey WC, Benowitz NL, Curry SJ et al. *Treating Tobacco Use and Dependence: 2008 Update. Clinical Practice Guideline.* Rockville, MD: U.S. Department of Health and Human Services, Public Health Service, 2008.

8. Reddy SS, Shaik Hyder Ali KH. Estimation of nicotine content in popular Indian brands of smoking and chewing tobacco products. *Indian J Dent Res* 2008;19:88–91.

9. Hughes JR, Stead LF, Lancaster T. Antidepressants for smoking cessation. *Cochrane Database Syst Rev* 2007;(1):CD000031.

10. Mooney ME, Sofuoglu M. Bupropion for the treatment of nicotine withdrawal and craving. *Expert Rev Neurother* 2006;6:965–81.

11. Spina E, Trifirò G, Caraci F. Clinically significant drug interactions with newer antidepressants. *CNS Drugs* 2012;26(1):39–67.

12. Jimenez-Ruiz C, Berlin I, Hering T. Varenicline: A novel pharmacotherapy for smoking cessation. *Drugs* 2009;69:1319–38.

13. Aubin HJ, Luquiens A, Berlin I. Pharmacotherapy for smoking cessation: Pharmacological principles and clinical practice. *Br J Clin Pharmacol* 2014;77(2):324–36.

14. Cahill K, Stevens S, Perera R, Lancaster T. Pharmacological interventions for smoking cessation: An overview and network meta-analysis. *Cochrane Database Syst Rev* 2013, (5). Art. No.: CD009329. DOI: 10.1002/14651858.CD009329.pub2. Accessed on June 15, 2015.

# CHAPTER 6

# How to Develop a Tobacco Cessation Center

Rana J. Singh

**Objectives**

The major objectives are to

- Understand the need for establishing tobacco cessation services at all levels of health care delivery

- Understand the virtues of a good tobacco cessation center, which delivers comprehensive and affordable cessation services

**Skill Sets You Will Acquire**

You will be able to conceptualize

- The virtues of a tobacco cessation center
- Tobacco cessation in special situations

## INTRODUCTION

While it is important that all health care providers provide brief intervention for tobacco cessation as part of routine health care, dedicated tobacco cessation services should be established in different health care settings at the primary, secondary, and tertiary levels. Specialist care may be provided particularly to help people with more severe tobacco dependence. According to the 2009 Global Adult Tobacco Survey (GATS), out of the 275 million tobacco users in India, an estimated 36% attempted to quit using tobacco in the past 12 months.

Many of these people would benefit from support from a tobacco cessation service. Even if just 5% of them accessed such services, this would still mean treating around 5 million people a year in India—which is a huge public health challenge for the country.

Tobacco cessation services can be set up preferably in different departments of a hospital or a medical college, such as dental, medicine, surgery, ENT, psychiatry, community medicine, TB and chest diseases, pediatrics, and obstetrics and gynecology.[1]

A good tobacco cessation center is a professionally staffed clinic which provides quality, evidence-based care in a nonjudgmental, and supportive environment. It provides a combination of behavioral therapy and medication that has been proved to increase the chance of success in quitting permanently.[2]

Such a specialized setting can be run by a team consisting of a trained physician, a counselor and a social worker attendant. A trained nurse, pharmacist, or health worker can also provide counseling services. Additionally, the delivery of tobacco cessation services at primary or secondary health facilities requires a specific service area in the health facility and the availability of appropriate tools.

## SETTING UP A TOBACCO CESSATION CENTER

Virtues of a Tobacco Cessation Center

A good tobacco cessation center must fulfill the following requirements:

1. Professionals who care

2. Dedicated service area

3. Appropriate cessation tools

4. Comprehensive and affordable cessation plans

5. A well-designed referral system

In addition, such a center should also provide tobacco cessation services in special populations such as pregnant and lactating women, patients with mental illnesses, patients with tobacco-related diseases, and people with other comorbidities (e.g., TB, diabetes, HIV/AIDS).

*Professionals Who Care*
Staff working in the cessation center should approach each client/patient with dignity, understanding, and compassion. They are dedicated in their mission to work with and support each client/patient achieve the goal of quitting tobacco use. Their work includes helping patients understand the options available to them and to create a customized plan to help them on their journey toward quitting tobacco.

Further, they should be educated in both psychosocial as well as in pharmacological interventions. Staff should be sufficiently trained in counseling skills and retrained annually on the updated developments in the clinical practice of tobacco cessation.

*The current situation in India*: In India, tobacco cessation services both at the community and at the cessation center levels have yet to be fully evolved and have a long way to go before they can actually support tobacco users in quitting.

*Community cessation*: Primary health care providers in India have several roles to play in tobacco control, including assisting tobacco users in quitting. Despite the evidence on the effectiveness and cost-effectiveness of brief tobacco interventions, most primary care providers, especially those in low- and middle-income countries, do not routinely deliver these interventions.[3] The lack of knowledge and skills about tobacco and tobacco control is a major barrier to the provision of brief tobacco interventions.

*Clinic-based tobacco cessation*: In 2002, the WHO country office and the Ministry of Health and Family Welfare, Government of India, set up tobacco cessation clinics (TCCs) to provide the first formal tobacco cessation intervention. Thirteen clinics were set up in oncology, cardiology, psychiatry, and surgery departments and in NGO settings, and later expanded to nineteen. The main objectives of this initiative were to evolve treatment approaches for the management of smoking and smokeless tobacco dependence, to generate experience in the implementation of these interventions, and to study the feasibility of implementing these interventions on a large scale. In the first 5 years, 34,741 cases were registered at these clinics and baseline information was recorded for 23,320 cases. Only behavioral strategies were employed in 69% of the cases; and pharmacotherapy, primarily bupropion and nicotine gum were used in 31% along with behavioral counseling. At 6 weeks, 14% had quit and 22% had reduced their tobacco intake by 50% or more. Younger male patients, users of smokeless forms of tobacco, and those receiving a combination of pharmacotherapy and behavioral counseling had relatively better outcomes at 3, 6, and 9 months. The longer the patients remained in follow-up, the greater the chances of quitting successfully or reducing consumption.[4] This model of service has several limitations, which need to be overcome in a diverse country such as India. These include

- These TCCs covered a very small number of the tobacco-user population

- Most of the clinics were predominantly urban

- Follow-up varied in different TCCs

- Use of tobacco quitting services was very limited among young people

Thus, to ensure that tobacco cessation becomes an integral part of health care in the Indian settings, the problems and recommendations listed in Table 6.1 need to be considered.

Every effort should be made to ensure that tobacco cessation services are available in all health care facilities to maximize the chances of continued counseling and successful quit attempts. A study by Cherian Varghese et al. in 2012 on setting up tobacco cessation services in India concluded that it is possible to establish effective tobacco cessation services in diverse health settings with optimal use of existing infrastructure and minimal support.[5]

*Dedicated Service Area*

The hallmark of a good cessation counseling is privacy. Ideally, enough space should be available for the patient and the counselor to sit comfortably during the counseling sessions. Comfort, privacy, and an interruption- and noise-free atmosphere are essential for a better rapport between the client and the therapist. Preferably, an exclusive room or a designated area adequately separated should be made available for Tobacco Cessation Center (TCC) and counseling. However, the lack of a separate space should not prevent health care professionals from counseling the patient. At least, a brief intervention should be provided at OPD/indoor/lab area/pharmacy area. While managing groups of people to quit smoking, a suitably large enough area needs to be available to enable some 20 people to be seated in a circle.

TABLE 6.1 Recommendations for Staffing of Tobacco Cessation Services in Indian Health Care Settings

| S. no. | Type of Health Center | Main Staffing Issues | Recommendations |
|---|---|---|---|
| 1 | PHC/CHC/City hospitals | Adequate availability of health care professionals (HCPs) | Frontline HCPs should be trained in brief interventions and those involved in cessation services should be trained in intensive counseling. |
| 2 | PHC/CHC/City hospitals | Inadequate availability of health personnel | When time permits, intensive counseling may be provided. Otherwise, brief intervention may be provided. Groups counseling is another possibility where staff time is limited. |
| 3 | Tertiary care hospitals (medical and dental colleges) | Multitasking nature of jobs of health professionals | Clinical staff of relevant departments should be trained in brief interventions and those involved in cessation services should be trained in intensive counseling. |
| 4 | Tertiary care hospitals (medical and dental colleges) | Specific nature of jobs of health professionals | A dedicated Tobacco Cessation Center along with a referral system in place. |
| 5 | Integrated Counseling and Testing Center (ICTC) available | Staff trained in patient counseling already available | The ICTC counselor should be trained in tobacco cessation and nominated as the nodal person for behavioral service delivery. All other staff should be trained in brief interventions. |
| 6 | TB microscopic center (no ICTC/ANC Clinic/NCD Clinic) | Adequate availability of health professionals | Training of relevant HCPs in brief interventions: 1–2 staff or an NCD paramedic should be designated the nodal person for behavioral service delivery |
| 7 | Subcenter | Health worker available | Training in brief interventions. |
| 8 | Special clinics/hospitals (MCH clinics, mental hospitals, heart institutes | Adequate staff available | Relevant staff should be trained in brief interventions and those involved in cessation services must be trained in intensive counseling. |
| 9 | Workplace health care | Adequate staff available | Identified staff should be trained in brief and/or intensive behavioral interventions. |

*Appropriate Cessation Tools*

Client education materials, including audiovisual displays, dependence assessment tools, a carbon monoxide monitor, and so on, are important tools for a TCC clinic. The following materials should be available for the purpose of client education and recording cessation-related information:

1. Fagerström test questionnaire

2. Patient education posters

3. Flip books/charts for counseling

4. Patient education materials (take away message)

5. Counseling register

6. Follow-up register

7. Patient case history record

8. Monthly activity reporting format

9. Tobacco cessation intervention (TCI) card for cessation among people with tobacco-related comorbidities

For physical examination, the following TCC-specific equipment should be provided:

*Carbon monoxide (CO) monitor (Smokerlyzer)*: CO is easily measured through the breath test using a CO monitor: It is quick to carry out, and provides a cost-effective means of validating the smoking status of a significant number of clients, and it is also noninvasive.[6] It measures the amount of carbon monoxide in the breath (ppm), which is an indirect measure of blood carboxyhemoglobin (%COHb), which is the level of CO in the blood (Figure 6.1).

*Spirometer*: A spirometer is an apparatus that measures the volume of the air inspired and expired by the lungs. It measures ventilation,

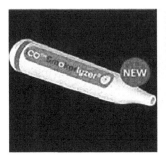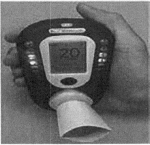

FIGURE 6.1    Examples of carbon monoxide monitors.

the movement of air into and out of the lungs. Performing a spirometry test and providing information on pulmonary function may increase the awareness of the effect of smoking among smokers who are asymptomatic or have fewer symptoms, and provide further motivation in their attempt to quit.[7] If airflow obstruction is present (as evidenced by a reduction in [FEV] 1.0), this can be shown to patients as an indicator of the damage induced to their lungs by smoking. Based on a spirometer, lung age can also be calculated and provided to the patient. Telling a 35-year-old male smoker that his lung function is similar to that predicted for a 70 year old is likely to be more of an eye-opener than telling him that his FEV 1.0 is 77% of the predicted figure (Figure 6.2).

What is lung age? The accompanying predictive formula was derived from normal Caucasian subjects (Crapo RO 1981). It allows

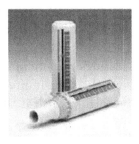

FIGURE 6.2    Commonly used spirometer.

you to enter the patient's gender, height, and measured FEV1.0, then derive the age for which that FEV1.0 value is 100% predicted. So, the lung age = (2,87 × height in inches) − (31,25 × observed FEV1) − 39,375.

*Sphygmomanometer*: Used to measure blood pressure.

*Stethoscope*: Used to examine chest and heart sounds.

The general items which are important to furnish a TCC:

1. Table and chair
2. Curtains to ensure privacy
3. Light and fan
4. Telephone/mobile service for follow-up
5. Computer for AV display and the recording of patient information and reporting

## Tobacco Cessation Medications
The most important and commonly used medications that should be in place at a cessation facility/TCC include:

*Nicotine replacement therapy (NRT)*: In the Indian scenario, the NRTs which can be made available at TCCs are nicotine gums (2 and 4 mg) and nicotine patch 21 mg.

*Non-nicotine replacement therapy*: This group of drugs includes antidepressants like bupropion (150 mg) and nortriptyline (25 mg) and nicotine receptor partial agonist drugs: varenicline, available in 0.5 and 1.0 mg.

### A Comprehensive and Affordable Cessation Plan
A comprehensive cessation treatment plan addressing all cessation needs includes individual, group, and telephone counseling and

the availability of approved cessation medication. The box that follows shows some important facts about cessation counseling:
The plan must include follow-up calls and visits, as needed. It can be supported by a helpline, quitline, or text-messaging support where possible.

*A Good Referral System*
The presence of a good inter- and intra-institutional referral system for patients/clients requiring referral is another important factor to ensure the success of cessation facilities/cessation centers.

*Inter-institutional referral*: Tobacco users requiring intensive counseling, specialized care, or pharmacotherapy may be referred from field-level institutes like subcenters, PHCs, and CHCs to city or tertiary hospitals as well as from workplaces.

*Intra-institutional referral*: All clinical departments including specialized clinics must ask for history of tobacco use, make an offer of support to quit, and refer those patients that are interested in quitting to the TCC within the hospital for tobacco cessation treatment.

## TOBACCO CESSATION IN SPECIAL SITUATIONS

The cessation facilities/centers must also address the following special situations.[9]

### Pregnant and Lactating Females

Women who use tobacco during pregnancy and breastfeeding should be strongly advised against it. They should be asked to quit using the behavioral strategies that were mentioned earlier, to deal with withdrawal. However, if they are unable to quit just by behavior counseling, then the use of NRT may be considered. Pregnant and breastfeeding women who opt for NRT should be advised to use shorter acting products to minimize overnight fetal exposure to nicotine, for example, nicotine gum. If a patch is judged to be the most appropriate NRT product, then the pregnant woman should remove it overnight.[10]

## Patients with Tobacco-Related Diseases

This is a group where tobacco cessation is an urgent clinical need, as continued tobacco use greatly increases the risk of further illness. All pharmacotherapy can be considered. Nicotine patches have been studied extensively in patients with stable CVD and have been shown to be safe. There is evidence that bupropion and varenicline can increase cessation rates in chronic tobacco users with mild-to-moderate chronic obstructive pulmonary disease and CVD.[11] People with tobacco-related diseases may benefit from a multidisciplinary care plan. Intensive behavioral therapy is more effective and should be delivered when possible.

---

**FACTS ABOUT CESSATION COUNSELING**

For individual treatment, the required competencies include:

- Cessation counseling and medications are effective in increasing quit rates when used separately and even more effective when used together
- Even brief cessation advice by health care providers is effective, and should be offered to every patient
- The effectiveness of cessation counseling increases with the intensity of the counseling, including the length and number of counseling sessions
- Telephone quitline counseling and text messaging increase quit rates, and are effective with diverse populations, and have a broad outreach[8]

---

## Patients with Mental Illness

Patients with mental health problems have higher rates of smoking/tobacco use and are prone to serious health problems on account of both mental illness and tobacco use. The treatment of mental illness needs to be monitored carefully during tobacco cessation.

### Persons with Substance Use Disorders

Smoking and tobacco use is common in persons with substance-use disorders. Tobacco cessation must be offered to such persons in inpatient and outpatient settings.

### Tobacco Users with Weight Gain Apprehension

Some tobacco users are apprehensive about quitting tobacco as it may lead to weight gain. Such persons should first be reassured that weight gain can be attenuated by eating a proper diet and exercise. Typically, the benefits of stopping smoking outweigh the risks of some weight gain; however, particular attention should be given to those who are already overweight or obese. Tobacco cessation medications can delay weight gain. Continuing reassurance and support are vital for successful quitting.

## STRENGTHENING HEALTH SYSTEMS FOR TREATING TOBACCO DEPENDENCE IN PRIMARY CARE

The above package of tobacco cessation services at all levels will not be successful until health systems for treating tobacco dependence in primary care settings are strengthened. Integration of brief tobacco interventions (brief advice) into primary care and organizational smoke-free policies are critical first steps. A tobacco cessation policy, a dedicated cessation area and staff, appropriate cessation tools, and a comprehensive cessation plan can only be established under a strengthened health system. The training of policy makers, primary care service managers, and primary care providers, based on the understanding that the whole health care system needs to function well, and all health system actors should improve their skills and play a better role to improve the integrated delivery of brief tobacco interventions in primary care.[12]

## CONCLUSION

Tobacco cessation is a dynamic process that occurs over time rather than as a single event, and should be an integral part of health care interventions. While India has developed tobacco control legislation which prohibits smoking at public places; has banned the sale of tobacco products to minors; has banned any kind of tobacco advertisement, promotion, and sponsorships; and has mandated the display of specified health warnings, there is still an urgent need for scale-up of the establishment of tobacco cessation in both public and private sectors at all levels of health care delivery. These facilities need to ensure that the techniques used for tobacco cessation can be implemented cost-effectively.

**KEY MESSAGES**

- To support many of the 100 million tobacco users who want to quit in India, there is a need to establish tobacco cessation centers in different health care settings at the primary, secondary, and tertiary levels
- An ideal tobacco cessation center has the following virtues: caring professionals, dedicated service area, appropriate cessation tools, comprehensive and affordable cessation plan, and a well-designed referral system
- Cessation facilities should be well-equipped to deal with patients with special requirements and with special situations

## REFERENCES

1. Tobacco Cessation Centre, NIMHANS. 2009. Starting tobacco cessation services. Available at: http://www.nimhans.kar.nic.in/deaddiction/1221/pub/Starting_TCC_Services-Nimhans_2009.pdf.
2. Available at: http://www.swgeneral.com/outpatient-services/outpatient-clinics/tobacco-cessation-clinic/.
3. Strengthening health systems for treating tobacco dependence in primary care/Part III at Available at: http://www.who.int/tobacco/publications/building_capacity/training_package/treatingtobaccodependence/en/.
4. Murthy P, Saddaichha S. Tobacco cessation services in India: Recent developments and the need for expansion. *IJC* 2010;47(5);69–74. Available at: http://www.indianjcancer.com/article.asp?issn=0019-509X;year=2010;volume=4 7;issue=5;spage=69;epage=74;aulast=Murthy.

5. Verghese C, Kaur J, Desai NG et al. Initiating tobacco cessation services in India: Challenges and opportunities. *WHO South-East Asia J Public Health* 2012;1(2):159–68.
6. Bittoun R. Carbon monoxide meter: The essential clinical tool—the "stethoscope"—of smoking cessation. *J Smok Cessat* 2008;3(2):69–70. DOI: 10.1375/jsc.3.3.69.
7. Irizar-Aramburu MI, Martínez-Eizaguirre JM, Pacheco-Bravo P et al. Effectiveness of spirometry as a motivational tool for smoking cessation. *BMC Fam Pract* 2013;14:185.
8. Fiore MC, Jaen CR, Baker TB et al. *Treating Tobacco Use and Dependence: 2008 Update. Clinical Practice Guideline.* Rockville, MD: Centers for Disease Control and Prevention, U.S. Department of Health and Human Services, 2008. Available at: http://www.ahrq.gov/professionals/clinicians-providers/guidelines-recommendations/tobacco/index.html#Clinic. Accessed January 21, 2014.
9. Tobacco Dependence Treatment Guidelines. *National Tobacco Control Programme (NTCP).* Government of India, 2011.
10. Benowitz N, Dempsey D. Pharmacotherapy for smoking cessation during pregnancy. *Nicotine Tob Res* 2004;6(Suppl 2):S189–202.
11. Joseph AM, Fu SS. Smoking cessation for patients with cardiovascular disease: What is the best approach? *Am Jl Cardiovasc Drugs* 2003;3(5):339–49.
12. WHO. Strengthening health systems for treating tobacco dependence in primary care. 2013 Available at: https://extranet.who.int/iris/restricted/bitstream/10665/84388/1/9789241505413_eng_Part-I_policy_makers.pdf.

# CHAPTER 7

# Patient Follow-Up

## Vikrant Mohanty

### Objectives

The major objectives are to

- Understand the need for follow-up during clinical interaction
- Structure follow-up visits and appropriately record suitable information
- Understand the barriers to follow-up

### Skill Sets You Will Acquire

You will be able to conceptualize

- The idea behind patient follow-up after imparting an intervention
- How to follow-up with a tobacco user after counseling/intervention
- The need to follow-up with your clients and also the barriers to follow-up

## INTRODUCTION

Tobacco dependence is a chronic disease that often requires repeated intervention and multiple attempts to quit. Effective treatments exist, however, that can significantly increase the rate of long-term abstinence. It is essential that clinicians and health care delivery systems consistently identify and document tobacco-use status, treat every user seen in a health care setting, and provide adequate support through follow-up and render continuity of care.[1]

The relapsing nature of tobacco dependence makes it mandatory for follow-up with the patients. The relapse rate of tobacco smoking after a quitting attempt is the greatest in the first few weeks, then decreases rapidly over time, and the longer the period of abstinence, the lower the rate of relapse.[2] Hence, managing timely follow-up would assist in long-term tobacco abstinence. Follow-up is a key step during intensive intervention with or without pharmacotherapy.

The benefits of follow-up include:

1. It provides repeated opportunity for tobacco cessation advice and support

2. It improves the likelihood of quitting

3. It ensures commitment for the change (quitting)

4. It ensures continuity of care and reinforces complete abstinence from tobacco

When scheduling follow-up treatment, the following factors should be considered:

a. Level of nicotine dependence

b. Comorbidities (e.g., mental illness)

c. History of unsuccessful quit attempts

d. Other factors including the availability of health professionals and patients, combined with follow-up with scheduled visits for other treatment, and logistics (e.g., patients able to attend follow-up)

Follow-up sessions should be negotiated with patients. Record patient contact information including mobile numbers in the Tobacco Cessation Center (TCC) register. Patients can be reminded of follow-up sessions via mobile text messages, telephonic conversation, or frontline health workers such as an accredited social health activist (ASHA) or an auxiliary nurse midwife (ANM).

Ensure that the first follow-up is within the first 2 weeks of the quit date and the second one is within the first 1 month of quitting. The subsequent follow-ups could be scheduled through a monthly contact for the next 6 months, which is ideal, or can be spaced out to 3-month intervals during the course.[3] It is preferable to conduct at least 3–4 follow-up sessions in person, and if there are constraints, then follow-up can be scheduled through telephone or home visits by health workers.

## STEPS FOR FOLLOW-UP TREATMENT

1. Follow-up is a planned professional aspect of the cessation intervention. It should be initiated preferably within 2 weeks of the quit date.

2. The concerned health care professional should be available for the follow-up visit also.

3. Data recording should include[5]:

    a. Tobacco-use analysis (abstinence/regular use/reduced use/relapse). For example, with smoking we might ask "Since your last visit have you smoked at all?"

       – No, not a single puff

       – Yes, just a few puffs

- Yes, 1–5 cigarettes

- Yes, more than 5 cigarettes (If they choose this answer, you might also like to ask how many cigarettes they are smoking a day)

b. Carbon monoxide levels in expired breath (if CO monitor is available).

c. Status of craving and other tobacco withdrawal symptoms and management strategy: The withdrawal symptoms vary from client to client. It is important to inform the client about common withdrawal symptoms and coping mechanisms at the beginning of the quit attempt.

d. Relapse prevention: Many tobacco users undergo relapse before finally reaching abstinence and can be considered as part of the process. It is important to assess every episode of relapse and understand the various triggers.

4. In case of complete abstinence, it is the health professional's responsibility to applaud the patient's efforts and congratulate them on their success. It is important to discuss the strategies used by the patient to overcome the withdrawal symptoms and triggers.

They should be classified and recorded as "enablers" and "detractors." The various enabling factors which have promoted complete abstinence could be fresh breath, better taste, and the ability to carry out daily work in a better way. The various detractors that have forced a lapse or relapse can be: Being around tobacco users, stressful situations, drinking coffee or an alcoholic beverage, and feeling bored.

5. If the client has relapsed (i.e., back to regular tobacco use) or has had certain "slips or lapses" during the period, the health professional must assess the situation. Relapse does not indicate a failure of the intervention or lack of motivation from the patient. It is an opportunity for the health care

professional to understand the strategies implemented and to reassess various situations that might encourage the relapse.

First, the health professional must assess the precise situation and various factors that led to this lapse during that point of time. Then, it is important to thread all the series of events that led to the lapse and also understand the behavior following these lapses. If the repeated lapses along with a lack of regret among the users are reinforced, it becomes more difficult for the patient to quit or attend follow-up.

6. Follow-up visits should also assess the status of pharmacotherapy, and the necessary reinforcement should be provided. Any adverse drug reactions (ADRs) should be recorded during follow-up sessions. In the case of any ADRs, first assess the extent of reactions as compared to standard drug interactions, and based on this information, either change the medication or discontinue it if needed.

7. Every follow-up visit should be structured and clear, strongly reinforcing the need for complete abstinence. The physician/health worker should be well-versed with the patient's history and personalize the feedback in a comprehensive and realistic manner.

8. The health care professional must continue to motivate, reinforce, and encourage maintenance of complete abstinence and schedule the next visit. The next visit should be scheduled within the completion of the first month and then, preferably, once every month until 6 months. Long-term follow-up can be performed at 12 months and done by telephone, or can be aligned with the next personal visit to the health center.

9. If follow-up is not possible in the clinic, arrange group counseling sessions in the community if the clients are comfortable, or arrange home visits by the health workers.

10. The client should be made aware of whom to contact, location of the clinic, and the timing. In case there is a relapse, withdrawal symptoms, or adverse drug reactions during the period, they should also be told whom to contact in such cases.

11. Unsuccessful contacts and those lost to follow-up: Two attempts by phone (ideally on different days and different times) should be made to contact all clients who have been newly referred to the service, or who have missed a scheduled consultation. Following the second unsuccessful attempt, a text, email, or letter should be sent to the client to inform them that the service has been unable to make contact and information for reentering the service should be provided. In the case of 1-, 3-, and 12-month calls to assess quit status, the facility will ask patients to advise the service of their status.[6]

**FOLLOW-UP SESSION SCHEDULE**
- Opening remarks and assess current smoking status
- If abstinent, congratulate and remind and motivate the patient
- If there is a relapse or lapse, recognize and discuss
- Review medication status and reassess
- Review medical treatment in line with cessation
- Formulate short-term, realistic, and achievable goals
- Schedule next appointment and note closing remarks

**KEY MESSAGES**
- Reinforce the potential benefits of change
- Bolster self-efficacy for behavior change
- Take the opportunity to encourage success
- Provide realistic and short-term achievable goals

## RECORD KEEPING DURING FOLLOW-UP

1. Record keeping during follow-up, whether it is by a personal visit or by telephone, is essential to completely understanding the patient.

2. Record keeping should be structured, and physicians or health workers should be adequately trained and repeatedly evaluated for compliance.

3. Record keeping during follow-up visits allows us to understand:

   • Tobacco use following the session (abstinence/regular use/reduced use/relapse).

   • Measurement of cravings and other withdrawal symptoms and their management—Cravings can result from triggers, which may include any of the following: Like being around tobacco users, starting the day fresh, feeling stressed, traveling, drinking coffee or tea or enjoying a meal or drinking an alcoholic beverage, and feeling bored. Cravings and other withdrawal symptoms can be measured using simple questionnaires such as the Mood and Physical Symptom Scale.[8] The withdrawal symptoms will vary from client to client. It is important to inform the client about the common withdrawal symptoms and coping mechanisms prior to the first visit (see Chapter 3).

   • Relapse prevention: Relapse is common, and does not imply a personal failure. If tobacco use has occurred; assess the environment for triggers and also motivate for recommitment to total abstinence. Review the circumstances that caused the lapse and encourage the client to either avoid or refrain from exposing themselves to such situations and to use the lapse as a learning experience.[3-5]

## BARRIERS TO FOLLOW-UP[4–7]

The following is a list of barriers to follow-up and abstinence. Discuss these with your patient as appropriate.

- The myth that tobacco use is a "stress buster"
- Lack of confidence in the treatment system and its effectiveness
- Stigmatization and fear of treatment being similar to psychiatric care
- Denial that they need help and can refrain from tobacco use at any point of time
- Lack of financial resources
- Distance from health care facility and other logistic issues
- Privacy concerns
- Lack of time
- Poorly trained professionals
- Lack of treatment availability
- Negative social support (e.g., unsupportive friends or family)
- High prevalence and acceptability among peers and vulnerable communities

Regular follow-up is important for long-term abstinence. During the initial session, the client should be made aware of the need for regular follow-up and the role it plays in maintaining a tobacco-free life.

## REFERENCES

1. Fiore MC et al. *Treating Tobacco Use and Dependence: 2008 Update. Clinical Practice Guideline.* Rockville, MD: U.S. Department of Health and Human Services. Public Health Service. May 2008.

2. Vangeli E et al. Predictors of attempts to stop smoking and their success in adult general population samples: A systematic review. *Addiction* 2011;106(12):2110–21.
3. World Health Organization. *Helping People Quit Tobacco: A Manual for Doctor and Dentists*. Geneva: WHO, 2010.
4. NIMHANS. Starting Tobacco Cessation Clinic. Tobacco Cessation Center, NIMHANS with support from the WHO Country Office and Ministry of Health and Family Welfare, Government of India, 2009.
5. Manual for Tobacco Cessation. Directorate General of Health Services. Ministry of Health and Family Welfare. Government of India. November 2005.
6. National Standard for Tobacco Cessation Support Program. HSE Tobacco Control Framework Implementation Group. March 2013.
7. Twyman L, Bonevski B, Paul C et al. Perceived barriers to smoking cessation in selected vulnerable groups: A systematic review of the qualitative and quantitative literature. *BMJ Open* 2014;2(4):1–15.
8. West R, Hajek P. Evaluation of the mood and physical symptoms scale (MPSS) to assess cigarette withdrawal. *Psychopharmacology (Berl)* 2004, 177:195–9.

# CHAPTER 8

# Evaluation of Cessation Practices

Rakesh Gupta

**Objectives**

The major objective is to

- Describe the methods for evaluating a tobacco cessation service

**Skill Sets You Will Acquire**

You will be able to conceptualize

- Basic knowledge on evaluating tobacco cessation services

## INTRODUCTION

To assess tobacco-use prevention and control efforts adequately, we will usually need to supplement available data with data collected to answer specific evaluation questions. Along with collection of data on knowledge, attitudes, behaviors, and environmental indicators, we also need to collect project planning and implementation information to document and measure the effectiveness of an intervention, including its policy and media efforts.

## WHY EVALUATE TOBACCO PREVENTION AND CONTROL INTERVENTIONS?

There are many reasons for evaluating tobacco prevention and control interventions:

- To monitor progress toward the desired goals

- To demonstrate that a particular tobacco control program or activity is effective

- To determine whether intervention components are producing the desired effects

- To permit comparisons among groups, particularly among populations with disproportionately high tobacco use and adverse health effects

- To learn how to improve existing programs

- To ensure that only effective programs are maintained and resources are not wasted on ineffective programs

The Public Health Service (PHS) guidelines for treating tobacco use and dependence identify five key processes and six structures that have evidence indicating the need for raising the rate of smoking cessation in a tobacco cessation center. A tobacco cessation service can be evaluated by using the checklist shown in Table 8.1.[1]

Smoking cessation outcomes should be recorded at all follow-up sessions (see "How can abstinence be assessed?")

TABLE 8.1  Tobacco Cessation Structure of Care Checklist

| S. no. | PHS Recommendations Systems | 25-Item Checklist Survey for Health Care Systems |
|---|---|---|
| 1. | Every clinic should implement a tobacco-user identification system | **Identifying smokers**<br>1. Is there a system in place (e.g., part of vital signs) to ask about smoking at every visit in primary care?<br>2. Is there a system in place (e.g., part of vital signs) to ask about smoking at every visit in other clinics (e.g., subspecialty clinics, dental, etc.)?<br>3. Do the people assessing smoking status routinely refer smokers for further treatment?<br>4. Are there reminders (e.g., Post-it notes) for providers when a smoker is identified?<br>5. Is performance of the screening system monitored on a regular basis?<br>6. Is data on smoking status stored in a database where it can be accessed later? |
| 2. | All health care systems should provide education, resources, and feedback to promote provider interventions | **Provider intervention**<br>7. Are providers trained on smoking cessation on a regular basis?<br>8. Are smoking cessation resources (e.g., kits, brochures) available in every exam room?<br>9. Is institutional performance at smoking cessation measured?<br>10. Are providers given feedback about their individual performance at smoking cessation on a regular basis? |
| 3. | Clinical sites should dedicate staff to provide tobacco-dependence treatment and assess the delivery of this treatment in staff performance evaluations | **Staff dedicated to smoking cessation**<br>11. Is someone identified as the tobacco-dependence coordinator for your facility?<br>12. Are the responsibilities of the tobacco-dependence coordinator clearly defined?<br>13. Is the performance of the tobacco-dependence coordinator measured on a regular basis?<br>14. Are the roles of each discipline defined with respect to smoking cessation? |

*(Continued)*

TABLE 8.1 (*Continued*)  Tobacco Cessation Structure of Care Checklist

| S. no. | PHS Recommendations Systems | 25-Item Checklist Survey for Health Care Systems |
|---|---|---|
| 4. | Hospitals should promote policies that support and provide tobacco-dependence services | **Hospital policies related to smoking cessation**<br>15. Is there a system in place to identify smokers on admission to the hospital?<br>16. Is there a clinician identified to provide smoking cessation counseling to all smokers after admission to the hospital?<br>17. Are all hospitalized patients who use tobacco offered tobacco-dependence treatment?<br>18. Are pharmacologic treatments for smoking cessation available to inpatients?<br>19. Are hospital staff educated regularly about smoking cessation? |
| 5. | Insurers should include tobacco-dependence treatments (both counseling and pharmacotherapy) as paid or covered services | **Services offered for smoking cessation**<br>20. Is there a smoking cessation clinic at your facility?<br>21. Is the waiting time for a smoking cessation clinic appointment 1 week, more or less?<br>22. Are smoking cessation medications routinely used by the smoking cessation clinic?<br>23. Can primary care providers prescribe smoking cessation medications? |
| 6. | Insurers should reimburse clinicians and specialists for delivery of effective tobacco-dependence treatments and include these interventions among the defined duties of clinicians | **Performance incentives for smoking cessation**<br>24. Are there incentives for primary care providers with respect to smoking cessation?<br>25. Are there incentives for other staff with respect to smoking cessation? |

*Source:* Gupta R et al. A hospital-based model in systems approach in tobacco treatment in LMICs. Poster presented at the *16th World Conference on Tobacco Or Health*, Abu Dhabi, UAE. Poster discussion session no. 56—Cessation Patterns and Pathways, 2015. Accessed on March 21, 2015. 2015. Available at: http://www.who.int/tobacco/quitting/summary_data/en/.

## HOW CAN ABSTINENCE BE ASSESSED?

Smoking abstinence can be assessed using a 7- and 30-day window. Participants should be contacted and asked these questions in the following order:

1. Have you smoked a cigarette, even a puff in the last 7 days?

   - Yes → They are not abstinent for 7 or 30 days (you are finished assessing abstinence).
   - No → Go to # 2

2. Have you used any other tobacco products in the last 7 days? (Note: Nicotine replacement products are not to be counted in this question.)

   - Yes → They are not abstinent for 7 or 30 days (you are finished assessing abstinence).
   - No → Go to # 3. They are considered abstinent for 7 days.

3. Have you smoked a cigarette, even a puff in the last 30 days?

   - Yes → They are not abstinent for 30 days (you are finished assessing abstinence).
   - No → Go to #4.

4. Have you used any other tobacco products in the last 30 days?

   - Yes → They are not abstinent for 30 days.
   - No → They are considered abstinent for 30 days.

## REFERENCES

1. Gupta R, Gupta P, Khan S, Soni N. A hospital-based model in systems approach in tobacco treatment in LMICs. Poster presented at the *16th World Conference on Tobacco Or Health*, Abu Dhabi, UAE. Poster discussion session no. 56—Cessation Patterns and Pathways, 2015. Accessed on March 21, 2015. Available at: http://www.who.int/tobacco/quitting/summary_data/en/.

# CHAPTER 9

# Frequently Asked Questions

**What is NRT?**

NRT is an abbreviation for nicotine replacement therapy. Only nicotine gum is available on the Indian market. Other forms of nicotine are lozenges, patches, inhalers, sublingual tablets, and so on.

**Why replace nicotine from tobacco products with nicotine in NRT?**

Nicotine is the addictive chemical in tobacco products that makes a tobacco user dependent. It takes only seven seconds to reach the brain when inhaled from a smoking tobacco product (cigarette/bidi/hookah) and makes the user become addictive very quickly. Nicotine without carcinogens and other toxic chemicals of tobacco products that kill their users, help patients wean off the addiction while protecting them fully.

**Why use nicotine after stopping tobacco use? Isn't nicotine what a patient wants to give up?**

If sudden stopping (cold turkey) works for someone, it is a good enough reason for not starting NRT. However, NRT increases the odds of quitting tobacco use by around 60% compared to placebo. It reduces cravings and dampens the withdrawal symptoms such as irritability, anxiety, depression, and restlessness. The likelihood of long-term addiction from NRT is very low.

### Isn't quitting really about willpower?

Self-control and determination are almost always needed to quit tobacco use and it is the sole mechanism in the case of cold turkey. But, only about 5% users can quit this way. The rest requires assistance through counseling and/or medicines including NRT to quit successfully and to stay quit. The quit rate observed by adopting such methodology averages to ~30%.

### While quitting gradually using nicotine replacement therapy, how do you get the best results?

NRT and tobacco products must not be used simultaneously to avoid the toxic side effects of nicotine overdose. Quitting by one of the two gradual methods (tapering or delaying) should take just about a week. By quitting on the set quit date, the patient can start with NRT. However, those who are less confident to do so, may be put on bupropion a week before to reduce their craving for nicotine but to stay firm about the set quit date.

### How long should you use NRT?

At least 6–8 weeks use of NRT is recommended for the best results. Not using NRT long enough is generally more of a problem than using NRT for too long. Tobacco users should use NRT for as long as they require to feel 100% sure that they can give up tobacco use. A period of 2 weeks without cravings, withdrawal symptoms, or strong temptations to smoke is sometimes used to assess if someone is ready to stop NRT. Nevertheless, building patients capabilities and skills to stay quit by eliminating the psychological triggers, and, therefore, the role of counseling should not be underestimated.

### If NRT did not work in the past, should it be used again?

Nicotine replacement is not a magic bullet to quit tobacco use. Quitting tobacco use generally takes several attempts, with or without medications. Previous unsuccessful attempts to quit with NRT may be a result of an underdose. On the other hand, sometimes people genuinely do not find NRT very helpful. Patients may want to consider using prescription medications such as varenicline or bupropion instead.

### What are the solutions for some common NRT problems?

*Problem:* Oral products taste bad.

*Solution:* Nicotine has a hot, chili-like taste. People generally get used to the taste over a day or two. Switching brands for an acceptable flavor may help.

*Problem:* Hiccups or indigestion with gum.

*Solution:* The gum is to be chewed slowly, not too vigorously, alternating between chewing and holding the gum against the side of the mouth.

### Can minors use NRT?

Although NRT is safe for those under 18 years of age, it has not yet been proved to improve quit rates in adolescents. It may be considered only for dependent users, as it is much safer than tobacco use. Counseling is recommended prior to the consideration of the use of NRT. NRT is not to be used in those below 12 years of age.

### Does NRT cause cancer?

No. There are over 60 chemicals in cigarette smoke that cause cancer; none of these are in NRT. By quitting tobacco, you are greatly reducing your exposure to carcinogens and greatly lowering your risk of cancer.

### Does NRT cause weight gain?

No. While it is common to gain weight when quitting tobacco use, NRT will not add to it. Studies have shown that using nicotine gum can help minimize weight gain. Before quitting, make a plan to prevent weight gain. Drink plenty of water, exercise, and snack on healthy foods to keep off extra weight (but counsel that quitting should be given the priority over weight control).

### NRT is expensive. Can't I just use NRT when I think I need it the most?

No. The use of NRT is an investment indeed as it helps a patient to stay quit. One should not test himself/herself by deferring its use intermittently. Irregular use causes fluctuation in the level of nicotine in blood which causes a return of cravings, often worse than before. It is essential, therefore, to complete the whole course to ensure the patient is properly weaned off nicotine.

For best results, one needs to use the right amount of the NRT product for the right length of time by following the instructions given on the package. Asking a doctor or a pharmacist for more information and NRT prescription is the better course.

### Which patients who smoke are candidates for bupropion?

Bupropion could be offered to all smokers except those with contraindications. However, its use is recommended in:

- Smokers with symptoms of depression or anxiety
- History of intolerance or failure of NRT
- Smokers with recent myocardial infarction or other coronary syndrome
- Patients with concerns about weight gain
- Case of patient preference

### Why is smoking allowed during the first week of treatment with bupropion and varenicline?

Approximately 1 week of treatment is required to achieve steady-state blood levels of bupropion and varenicline for therapeutic action. As the half-life of these drugs is around "1 day," it will take at least five "half-life time," that is, 5 days to achieve a steady plasma level. Therefore, it is better to stop quitting after therapy for 1 week which would reduce withdrawal symptoms, especially cravings. It also allows the patient to prepare mentally for quitting.

**When 150 mg tablets are not available, can I take half of a 300 mg tablet?**

No. The tablet is enteric coated. Breaking into two halves will defeat its purpose. It may affect taste and absorption of drug and cause gastrointestinal side effects.

**Do I need a medical prescription to buy tobacco cessation medication?**

If you are planning to buy nicotine, a prescription is not required. However, advice by a physician followed by the use of NRT is always more helpful. For other cessation medicines, a prescription is necessary as these are potentially harmful.

**Varenicline is very costly and, hence, unaffordable. Is there an alternative available?**

Yes, there are alternatives although varenicline is the most effective drug presently. Please consult your doctor for available options in the case of inability to afford varenicline.

**Can NRT and bupropion or varenicline be used in combination?**

While bupropion and NRT can be used simultaneously, the use of NRT with varenicline is unnecessary due to both the agnostic and antagonistic action of the latter. It blocks nicotine receptor sites along with elimination of craving due to its direct suppressive action on the brain.

# Index

## A

Accredited social health activist
    (ASHA), 87
ADRs, *see* Adverse drug reactions
Adverse drug reactions (ADRs), 89
ANM, *see* Auxiliary nurse midwife
ASHA, *see* Accredited social health
    activist
Auxiliary nurse midwife (ANM), 87

## B

Behavioral; *see also* Tobacco
        cessation intervention
    change theories, 5
    techniques, 53
Bidi smokers, 65; *see also* First-line
        agents
Bite and park method, 60
Bupropion
    candidates for, 104
    hydrochloride, 65; *see also* First-
        line agents
    with other drugs, 105
    smoking during treatment,
        104–105

## C

Carbon monoxide monitor, 77, 78
Carcinogens, 11

Cerebrovascular disease, 12
Cessation practice evaluation, 95
    abstinence assessment, 99
    cessation care checklist, 97–98
    reasons for, 96
Chronic obstructive pulmonary
        disease (COPD), 13
Chronic respiratory symptoms, 13
CI, *see* Confidence interval
Clonidine, 66; *see also* Second-line
        agents
Combination treatment, 65; *see also*
        First-line agents
Combined interventions, 53; *see also*
        Tobacco cessation
        intervention
Confidence interval (CI), 49
COPD, *see* Chronic obstructive
        pulmonary disease
Coping with urges/cravings, 50–51;
        *see also* Tobacco cessation
        intervention
Coronary heart disease, 12
Cravings, coping with, 50–51;
        *see also* Tobacco cessation
        intervention
Cue conditioning, 27

## D

Drug interactions, 66; *see also* First-
        line agents

## E

Evidence-based approaches, 42; *see also* Tobacco cessation intervention

## F

Face-to-face counseling, 49–50; *see also* Tobacco cessation intervention
First-line agents, 59; *see also* Tobacco cessation pharmacotherapy
  bidi smokers, 65
  bupropion hydrochloride, 65
  combination treatment, 65
  drug interactions with bupropion, 66
  nicotine gum, 60, 64
  nicotine patches, 64
  principles of NRT use, 60
  special precautions, 65–66
  varenicline tartrate, 66
5A's approach, 43; *see also* Tobacco cessation intervention
Five D's approach, 50; *see also* Tobacco cessation intervention
5R's, 44, 45; *see also* Tobacco cessation intervention
Follow-up, 85
  barriers to, 92
  benefits of, 86
  record keeping in, 91
  treatment, 87–90
  treatment scheduling, 86–87
4A's approach, 52; *see also* Tobacco cessation intervention
Frequently asked questions, 101–105

## G

GATS, *see* Global Adult Tobacco Survey

Global Adult Tobacco Survey (GATS), 72
GATS India survey, 4
Group counseling, 49; *see also* Tobacco cessation intervention

## H

HCPs, *see* Health care professionals
Health care professionals (HCPs), 4

## I

ICD-10, *see* International Classification of Diseases
International Classification of Diseases (ICD-10), 2
Internet interventions, 49; *see also* Tobacco cessation intervention

## M

Mental disorders, 25
MI, *see* Motivational Interviewing
Minimal clinical intervention, 42–44; *see also* Tobacco cessation intervention
Motivational Interviewing (MI), 41
MPOWER measures, 4

## N

nAChR complex, 28
nAChRs, *see* Nicotinic acetylcholine receptors
Nasal ciliary beat frequency, 16
NCDs, *see* Noncommunicable diseases
Nicotine, 17; *see also* First-line agents
  bite and park method, 60
  brain changes in nicotine dependence, 29

gum, 60, 64
-induced vasoconstriction, 13
patches, 64
reasons to replace, 101
rewarding effect of, 29
Nicotine replacement therapy (NRT),
    58, 101
  age group for, 103
  candidates for bupropion, 104
  combination with drugs, 105
  cost of, 104
  frequently asked questions,
    101–105
  nicotine usage after stopping
    tobacco, 101–102
  obtaining best results, 102
  recommended period of, 102
  solutions for NRT problems, 103
  unsuccessful, 103
  usage principles, 60
Nicotinic acetylcholine receptors
    (nAChRs), 28
Noncommunicable diseases (NCDs), 2
Nortriptyline, 67; see also Second-
    line agents
NRT, see Nicotine replacement
    therapy

P

PAHs, see Polycyclic aromatic
    hydrocarbons
PHS, see Public Health Service
Plans, responses, impulses, motives,
    evaluations (PRIME), 5;
    see also Tobacco cessation
    intervention
PRIME Theory of Motivation, 41
Polycyclic aromatic hydrocarbons
    (PAHs), 11
Practical counseling techniques, 50;
    see also Tobacco cessation
    intervention

PRIME, see Plans, responses,
    impulses, motives,
    evaluations
Public Health Service (PHS), 96

Q

Quitlines, 48; see also Tobacco
    cessation intervention

R

Relative risk (RR), 49
Reproduction-related
    complications, 13
RR, see Relative risk

S

SD, see Substance dependence
Secondhand smoke, 14–16
Second-line agents, 66; see also
    Tobacco cessation
    pharmacotherapy
  clonidine, 66
  nortriptyline, 67
Self-help materials, 44–46; see also
    Tobacco cessation
    intervention
SIDS, see Sudden infant death
    syndrome
Smokerlyzer, see Carbon monoxide
    monitor
Smoking, 14
  competency in behavioral support
    for stopping, 47–48
  -induced respiratory disease, 12
  text messages for smoking
    cessation, 49
Social support, 52–53; see also
    Tobacco cessation
    intervention
Sphygmomanometer, 79

Spirometer, 77, 78
Stages of Change Model, see Trans-
    Theoretical Model
Stethoscope, 79
Substance dependence (SD), 24
Sudden infant death syndrome
    (SIDS), 15
Sudden unexplained death in infancy
    (SUDI), 13
SUDI, see Sudden unexplained death
    in infancy

T

TD, see Tobacco dependence
Technology-based interventions, 49;
    see also Tobacco cessation
    intervention
Telephone counseling, 48; see also
    Tobacco cessation
    intervention
Thirdhand smoke, 16–17
Tobacco
    control approach, 2
    dependence, 86
    as leading causes of death, 3
    smoke, 14
Tobacco addiction theories, 23, 35
    behavioral conditioning, 31–33
    biological theories, 28–30
    learning and conditioning, 27–28
    primary care physicians
        knowledge about, 33–34
    psychodynamic theories, 26–27
    theories of tobacco dependence, 26
    tobacco dependence, 24–26
    tobacco withdrawal symptoms,
        30–31
Tobacco and health, 9, 20
    acute respiratory disease, 12–13
    adverse health consequences, 10
    benefits of quitting tobacco, 17–20
    cardiovascular disease, 12

chronic respiratory disease, 13
death rate, 9–10
diseases caused by tobacco, 11
health impact, 9
misconceptions about tobacco
    use, 17, 18
secondhand smoke, 14–16
smoking and respiratory disease, 12
thirdhand smoke, 16–17
tobacco and cancer, 11–12
tobacco and reproductive health,
    13–14
tobacco and smoke composition, 10
toxins in tobacco smoke, 10
Tobacco cessation; see also Tobacco
    cessation intervention
counseling, 46–48, 81
medication prescription, 105
in mental illness, 81
pregnant and lactating females, 80
self-control, 102
services, 72
in substance use disorders, 82
in tobacco-related diseases, 81
weight gain apprehension, 82
Tobacco Cessation Center (TCC), 2,
    71, 74, 82–83, 87
affordable cessation plan, 79–80
carbon monoxide monitor, 77, 78
cessation medications, 79
cessation tools, 77–79
dedicated service area, 75
good referral system, 80
in India, 73
professionals, 73–75
recommendations for staffing
    of, 76
setting up, 73
sphygmomanometer, 79
spiromometer, 77, 78
stethoscope, 79
strengthening health systems, 82
virtues of, 73

Tobacco cessation intervention
(TCI), 39, 53, 77
  behavioral techniques, 53
  case studies, 54–55
  cessation counseling, 46–48
  combined interventions, 53
  common roadblocks, 45
  conceptual framework, 40–42
  evidence-based approaches, 42
  face-to-face counseling, 49–50
  5A's approach, 43
  Five D's, 50
  5R's, 45
  4A's approach, 52
  group counseling, 49
  identifying triggers and danger
    situations, 51–52
  learning to cope with urge for
    tobacco, 50–51
  minimal clinical intervention,
    42–44
  practical counseling techniques, 50
  PRIME Theory of Motivation, 41
  providing basic information, 50
  relapse rates, 40
  required competencies for
    behavioral support,
    47–48
  self-help materials, 44–46
  social support, 52–53
  technology-based interventions, 49
  text messages, 49
  Trans-Theoretical Model, 40–41, 42
Tobacco cessation pharmacotherapy, 57
  adolescents, 67
  case study, 68
  effectiveness of different agents, 67
  factors in choice of medications, 59
  first-line agents, 59–66
  medications for tobacco cessation,
    61–63
  pregnancy, 67
  psychiatric comorbidity, 67
  second-line agents, 66–67
  special populations, 67
Tobacco dependence (TD), 24
  biological theories, 28–30
  biopsychosocial model of, 32
  brain change in nicotine
    dependence, 29
  cue conditioning, 27
  nAChR complex, 28
  process of, 25
  protective factors, 26
  psychodynamic theories, 26–27
  risk factors, 26
  theories of, 26
  theory of learning and
    conditioning, 27–28
  vicarious learning, 27
Tobacco-specific nitrosamines
  (TSNAs), 11, 17
Tobacco use, 1, 6
  behavioral change theories, 5
  counseling and pharmacotherapy, 5
  GATS India survey, 4
  MPOWER measure, 4
  tobacco cessation centers, 2
Trans-Theoretical Model, 40–41, 42;
  see also Tobacco cessation
  intervention
TSNAs, see Tobacco-specific
  nitrosamines

U

Urges, coping with, 50–51; see also
  Tobacco cessation
  intervention

V

Varenicline; see also First-line agents
  alternatives, 105
  combination with other
    drugs, 105

Varenicline (*Continued*)
    smoking during treatment, 104–105
    tartrate, 66
Ventral tegmental area (VTA), 29
Vicarious learning, 27
VTA, *see* Ventral tegmental area

W

Web-based interventions, 49;
      *see also* Tobacco cessation
      intervention
Withdrawal symptoms, 30–31

Printed in the United States
by Baker & Taylor Publisher Services